PSILOCYBIN MUSHROOMS BIBLE

The Complete Guide to Psilocybin Mushrooms, Safe Use, Health Benefits, History and How to Grow Magic Mushrooms by your own

By Tyler Barrett

PSILOCYBIN MUSHROOMS

The Complete Guide to Psilocybin Mushrooms, Safe Use, Health Benefits, Magic Effects, History and Identification Guide for Magic Psychedelic Mushrooms.

By Tyler Barrett

© Copyright 2020 by Tyler Barrett

All rights reserved.

This document is geared towards providing exact and reliable information with regards to the topic and issue covered. The publication is sold with the idea that the publisher is not required to render accounting, officially permitted, or otherwise, qualified services. If advice is necessary, legal or professional, a practiced individual in the profession should be ordered.

- From a Declaration of Principles which was accepted and approved equally by a Committee of the American Bar Association and a Committee of Publishers and Associations.

In no way is it legal to reproduce, duplicate, or transmit any part of this document in either electronic means or in printed format. Recording of this publication is strictly prohibited and any storage of this document is not allowed unless with written permission from the publisher. All rights reserved.

The information provided herein is stated to be truthful and consistent, in that any liability, in terms of inattention or otherwise, by any usage or abuse of any policies, processes, or directions contained within is the solitary and utter responsibility of the recipient reader. Under no circumstances will any legal responsibility or blame be held against the publisher for any reparation, damages, or monetary loss due to the information herein, either directly or indirectly.

Respective authors own all copyrights not held by the publisher.

The information herein is offered for informational purposes solely, and is universal as so. The presentation of the information is without contract or any type of guarantee assurance.

The trademarks that are used are without any consent, and the publication of the trademark is without permission or backing by the trademark owner. All trademarks and brands within this book are for clarifying purposes only and are the owned by the owners themselves, not affiliated with this document.

Disclaimer

All Erudition contained in this book is given for informational and educational purposes only. The author is not in any way accountable for any results or outcomes that emanate from using this material. Constructive attempts have been made to provide information that is both accurate and effective, but the author is not bound for the accuracy or use/misuse of information.

Foreword

First, I will like to thank you for taking the first step of trusting me and deciding to purchase/read this life transforming eBook. Thanks for spending your time and resources on this material. I can assure you of exact blueprint I lay bare in the information manual you are currently reading. It has transformed lives, and I strongly believe it will equally transform your life too. All the information I presented in this Do-It-Yourself is easy to digest and practice.

Contents

Chapter 1 135

Chapter 2 3

Chapter 3 8

Chapter 4 20

Chapter 5 31

Chapter 6 38

Chapter 7 47

Chapter 8 69

Chapter 9 87

Chapter 10 96

Conclusion 127

Chapter 1

Introduction

Psilocybin mushrooms (aka, "magic mushrooms" or "shrooms") are fungi containing psilocybin, a psychedelic compound that occurs naturally. More than 180 mushroom species contain psilocybin, or its psilocybin derivative. Psilocybin mushrooms have a long history of spiritual and religious use in Mesoamerican rituals and are one of the most popular recreational psychedelics in the United States and in Europe. In therapeutic settings, psilocybin mushrooms have been used to treat a range of ailments and disorders including cluster headaches, obsessive-compulsive disorders, anxiety, depression and addiction. While psilocybin mushrooms have been decriminalized in two North American cities (see "Legality" for details), they are currently illegal and listed as a Schedule I controlled substance in the United States. Nevertheless, the FDA and DEA have recently approved a number of small, highly controlled human studies on their potential for use in medical and psychiatric environments.

Psychedelic mushrooms have a longstanding, deep, and storied background among the many cultures that have used them historically. Today, they recognize the benefits of these strong little fungi in a big way. Research are currently under way across the United States and internationally on the extensive and multifarious use of psychoactive mushrooms. One such study, published in the Journal of Psychopharmacology, found that, a single dose of psilocybin produced substantial and enduring declines in depressed mood and anxiety along with increases in quality of life. In addition, the mystical and profound experiences experienced by so many since psilocybin entered the American psychedelic lexicon in the 1960s, are now beginning to be tested and explored in the mainstream medical sciences.

The findings are encouraging and convincing, and paint as a powerful healer a substantiated, optimistic, symbiotic picture of the mushrooms. Specifically, clinical trials that involve patients with life-threatening cancer have been, and are currently being, conducted in the United States and abroad. These trials are mainly aimed at understanding the effectiveness of high-dose psilocybin, administered in therapeutic environments, as a tool to reduce psychological stress and anxiety that often accompanies a life-threatening diagnosis. Until now, the results have been promising. Under double-blind conditions, it has not only been shown to reduce psychological distress symptoms among terminal patient groups by a single high dose of psilocybin; the effects have been substantial and enduring.

In addition, there is a growing body of research indicating that one of the reason psilocybin is so powerful is that it causes neuroplasticity. That is, the ability of the brain to learn and grow, and to change.

Chapter 2

Brief History of Psilocybin Mushroom Cultivation

At the period of R. Gordon Wasson's "rediscovery" in Mexico in the 1950's of the shamanic use of psilocybin-containing mushrooms, the science of mushroom cultivation was still very much in its infancy. Until then, Agaricusbisporus, the common white button mushroom, was the only species of mushroom under cultivation, at least in the West. The methods of cultivation used were more or less the same as those conceived in France during the 1st 7th century: Farmers gathered mycelium-rich soil from wilderness areas where the mushroom was found and moved it to horse manure rows in naturally climatized caves. This method was effective but since it used a raw, unpasteurized substrate, it left much to chance and the beds were often contaminated. These crude methods remained essentially unchanged until the 20th century, when a number of incremental improvements were discovered; finally setting the stage for the successful cultivation of Psilocybecubensis in the 1960s. At the end of the 1st eighth century, American mushroom grower and researcher William Falconer published a book entitled: "Mushrooms: How to grow them; a Practical Treatise on Mushroom Culture for Profit and Pleasure" , which compiled recent discoveries in Agaricus cultivation, and included a chapter on the advantages of a "casing layer."

The French mycologist Roger Heim was the first individual to successfully cultivate several species of Psilocybin in the late 1950s, using materials brought back with from his voyages. In Mexico, Gordon Wasson tested each species they were collecting on a variety of sterilized substrates to determine optimum conditions for fruiting. He found the best fruiting on cased, sterilized horse dung occurred with Psilocyberubensis. However, his work remained largely unknown to the wider world because of the relative obscurity of Psilocybe mushrooms and their powerful effects, along with the fact that Heim's writings were not translated into English for almost twenty years. In the latter part of the 1960s, a number of "underground" pamphlets and booklets were published describing the manufacture and cultivation of a variety of psychedelic drugs (many of which were still legal to possess at that time), including several species of Psilocybe mushrooms. However, the techniques described were either crudely presented or far too technical to use with much success for the average person, and many of the books gave the impression that perhaps even the authors themselves had not put their own methods to the test.

A new cultivation manual, The PsilocybeFanaticus Technique, was published in 1991, by an enterprising experimenter by the questionable name PsilocybeFanaticus. His book described a highly efficient and almost foolproof technique of cultivating Psilocybecubensis on brown rice and "cakes" with vermiculite in half-pint mason jars. While this method (as it came to be known, the "PF Tek") obviously borrowed a lot from its predecessors, it was unique in a number of important ways. The substrate used was first of all a mixture of moistened brown rice flour and vermiculite. Its open, airy structure has made it an ideal medium for fast and vigorous growth of the fungus, eliminating the need to shake or otherwise disturb the substrate after inoculation. It was also readily sterilized in a simple boiling water bath, avoiding the need for the pressure cooker, one of the more prohibitively expensive and hard to get pieces of equipment previously essential for mushroom cultivation. Second, a thin layer of pure, dry vermiculite covered the PF substratum which served as an effective barrier to contaminants during inoculation and incubation. This permitted open handling of the cultures without the need for glove boxes or careful sterile techniques. In this way, minimizing much of the risk of contamination eliminated yet another obstacle that had previously stymied many would-be growers. The PF Tek also eliminated the need for difficult and contamination-prone agar techniques by using an aqueous suspension of the spores as inoculum. Upon sterilization of the substratum, it was injected from a syringe containing a sterile spore solution at several locations. The pre-hydrated spores soon germinated across the jar at many locations, and rapid colonization of the substratum.

Instead of relying on a casing layer to promote fruiting, the PF substratum popped out of the jar as a solid "cake," which was then placed in a small chamber containing a thick underlay of moist perlite (an inert water-absorbing material used in horticulture) that served wick water in the cake as well as humidifying the atmosphere inside the chamber. The cakes soon fruited on their outer surfaces at many locations when placed beneath enough lighting. Combined with the rapid dissemination of information in the age of Internet newsgroups and blogs, the absolute simplicity of the PsilocybeFanaticus Technique created a whirlwind of new interest in the production of Psilocybe mushrooms and spawned a whole generation of amateur growers. Meanwhile, just as PsilocybeFanaticus perfected his methods, another innovative amateur mycologist, Rush Wayne, PhD, was quietly preparing for his own cultivation revolution. Wayne, a trained biochemist, had become interested in growing edible mushrooms at home, but he had been discouraged from trying by his familiarity with the complications of sterile culture work. That is, until he read an article in a journal describing the use of hydrogen peroxide ($H2O2$) in germination of orchid seeds. Apparently, the peroxide in the agar medium killed bacteria, yeasts, and fungal spores, while leaving the orchid itself unharmed, because orchids, like most multi-cell organisms, generate peroxidases, enzymes that catalyze the oxidation of compounds into peroxides. Wayne wondered if this method could be applied to work with mushroom culture, since mushroom-producing fungi also synthesize peroxidases. He carried out a long series of experiments on various fungi and media, using a variety of peroxide concentrations, and discovered that his hunch was correct: most species of mushrooms grew quite happily in the presence of hydrogen peroxide, while contaminant organisms did not. So long as the media were sterile to begin with, the presence of relatively low peroxide concentrations made the crops contamination-resistant for long periods of time, enabling them to be treated outdoors without advanced techniques or equipment.

Chemically it's simply water that contains an extra oxygen atom. As this makes it a relatively unstable molecule, the extra atom is released readily as a radical vine. Free radicals are highly reactive and bind quickly to nearby molecules which can then become free radicals themselves, starting a chain reaction. If this cascade occurs unchecked within a biological system, it generally leads to death by cells. Most multi-celled organisms, including fungi, produce hydrogen peroxide and peroxidase enzymes as a protective device against bacteria, yeasts and viruses. Further, fungi use peroxides and peroxidases to break down their food sources ' cell walls. Since most fungi produce peroxidases, hydrogen peroxide does not provide protection against living fungi, including molds from contaminants. It does nonetheless destroy spores. Therefore, as Wayne found, the application of peroxide to cultures effectively shielded them from all airborne contaminants as long as the medium was properly sterilized or pasteurized to begin with. Wayne's invention, without doubt, marked a true revolution for generalized techniques of mushroom cultivation. What the PF Tek does for cultivation of Psilocybecubensis, the "peroxide tek" does for cultivation of almost all mushroom-producing fungi species. A procedure that had only been open to professionals with special skills and expensive equipment has now been made available to anyone with a pressure cooker, "a few mason jars, and a clean kitchen counter. It is no exaggeration to say that the book that you hold in your hands would not have been published without the discovery and writings of Rush Wayne.

Chapter 3

What is a Mushroom?

Relatively few of us, at least not by choice, have anything to do with the fungi. That is just as much a cultural phenomenon as anything else. When most people think of mushrooms, they imagine either the bland and innocuous toppings on their pizza, or the exotic, ornate fairy tale and legend toadstools, the mere taste of which will drive one mad, if not kill him outright. Mushrooms are either fearful poisons or inoffensive vegetables for the vast majority of North Americans, and not worthy of much thought in either case. Even if you're in that tiny minority for whom mushrooms bring curiosity, wonder, and delight (possibly due to one or more Psilocybe species experiences), you've probably learned little to nothing about them in your high school or college biology classes. What is a mushroom, then? A mushroom is just one part of a mushroom and not something in itself, just like you and your left elbow are connected, but it can hardly be said to be the same thing. Strictly speaking, mushrooms are some of the fungi's reproductive structures, roughly equivalent to the flowers on an apple tree that contains the "seeds" of future trees. That being said, fungi are neither plant nor animal although they are related to both. Not surprisingly there has always been a lot of confusion swirling around these mysterious and secretive creatures being properly classified. Most of us tend to think of mushrooms and fungi as an odd plant variety, as they often spring up like plants from the ground and seem unable to stand up and walk (or dance or swim) around like we lucky animals can. This is the primary misconception that most of us have about the fungi, and the one you should dispense with immediately. So here it is fungi are not plants, and it is not like gardening that growing mushrooms do. Then again, fungi are not animals either, although they are far more closely related to animals than plants despite appearances. Plants, algae, and certain bacteria synthesize their own food from sunlight, carbon dioxide, and water and are thus known as autotrophs. All other organisms, including fungi, are heterotrophs, meaning they derive energy from plants, or plant-eating things (say, a fish), or things that eat plant-eating things (a bigger fish). However, that's pretty much where the animal-fungi similarities end.

What are Hallucinogenic?

Hallucinogens are drugs which alter people's perception and mood. "The molecular, pharmacological, and physiological basis for hallucinogenic behavior is not well known," according to the Drug Enforcement Administration (DEA). What is understood is that these drugs cause changes in perception, thinking, and mood. These changes have the potential to be either pleasant or extremely scary.

Hallucinogens affect brain regions and structures, the neurotransmitters, which are responsible for coordination, processes of thought, hearing, and sight.

Hallucinogens can be present in or synthetic or natural plants and substances. Some popular natural hallucinogenic substances include peyote, psilocybin and psilocyn, and dimethyltryptamine (DMT). LSD, or diethylamide lysergic acid, is made from lysergic acid which is naturally found. Synthetic hallucinogens include dimethoxyamphetamine (DOM), ecstasy (MDMA) and phencyclidine (PCP).

Effects of Hallucinogens:

Hallucinogens actuate physiological, tangible and mystic effects. They are likewise known for causing flashbacks, in any event, when the person never again uses the drug. The physiological effects include:

- elevated heart rate
- increased blood pressure
- dilated students
- sleeplessness and tremors
- lack of muscle coordination
- sparse, disfigured, indistinguishable discourse
- decreased attention to contact or agony
- convulsions
- coma; heart and lung failure

The tactile effects of hallucinogen use incorporate perceptual twists. For instance, one may "hear" shading or "see" music.

The clairvoyant or mental effects include:

- disorders of thought related with reality
- depression, uneasiness, neurosis
- violent behavior

- confusion, doubt, loss of control
- schizophrenic psychosis-like behavior
- flashbacks
- severe despondency

The most significant thing to recall about hallucinogens is that every person will respond diversely relying on body size, dose and hallucinogenic drug type. Hallucinogens are entirely unpredictable, hazardous drugs, and similarly as the drugs themselves are unpredictable, so are the flashbacks, which occur all the more regularly during times of pressure and appear "to occur all the more much of the time in more youthful people" as indicated by the DEA.

What about Dependence?

Some hallucinogens, such as LSD, are not considered physically addictive, as compulsive drug-seeking behavior is not produced. Yet chronic users of hallucinogens have become psychologically dependent. These drugs have become the focal point of the thoughts, emotions, activities and whole lives of people.

The increased tolerance users have for the drugs is even more dangerous than the psychological dependence on the hallucinogens. Regular use of LSD, mescaline, ketamine, and psilocybin was known to induce tolerance within a few short days, requiring increased doses to produce the person's previously achieved state of intoxication (or trip). The danger in this situation is not so much an overdose but the self-mutilation or rash decisions that lead to accidents that threaten life. Although few people, with the exception of users of toxic jimson weed, have overdosed to a hallucinogen, many people die each year from accidents while under the effects of LSD, PCP or other hallucinogens.

How Are Hallucinogens Working?

Albert Hofmann, a Swiss scientist who invented the hallucinogenic drug LSD, died yesterday. But the LSD trip is far from over as scientists are bringing clarity to how hallucinogens function.

Hallucinogens, also called psychedelics, alter a person's perception, mood and a slew of other mental processes. Hallucinogenic history dates back centuries since people around the world took the drugs to induce altered states for religious and spiritual purposes.

While LSD (lysergic acid diethylamide), mescaline, and other psychedelics have been studied in the past, research largely came to a halt in the 1960s following recreational drug abuse, with some work resuming in the 1990s. Now, a lot of studies rely on animal models like mice.

One human study published in Psychopharmacology revealed the active ingredient in hippie mushrooms, called psilocybin, elicited "mystical experiences" for participants that allegedly resulted in weeks-long changes in behavior. Nearly one-third of the participants had a bad trip, though, reporting they found the drug experience scary.

Research has suggested that hallucinogens do their work mainly in the cortex of the brain, where the drugs stimulate unique receptors called 5-HT2A receptors (2ARs), which are normally activated by serotonin.

"In order to function, [the cortex] absorbs different signals, such as glutamate signals and serotonin signals," said neuroscientist Stuart Sealfon of Mount Sinai School of Medicine in New York, "and what hallucinogens must do is interrupt this cycle so that sensory perception becomes altered by them." "What made hallucinogens possess unique properties?" Sealfon said.

Scientists once thought of receptors as "locks and keys," in which some drugs fit into a particular receptor as a key fit into a lock. The receptor would then turn on and signal other cellular molecules.

Yet, for hallucinogens, that is not the case. Sealfon's research and his colleagues published in the journal Neuron last year revealed that the serotonin-2A receptor has more than one "on" position.

"When a non-hallucinogen activates the receptor, one cell signaling pattern in the brain is caused that is not hallucinogenic," Sealfon told LiveScience. "When a hallucinogen turns on this receptor, the receptor we infer has to go into a different position and that leads to a different pattern in cell responses and is what makes the hallucinogen have its unique effect." Psychedelics, also known as psychedelic drugs, hallucinogenic or hallucinogenic drugs, are chemical substances that induce hallucinations and other sensory disturbances. Lysergic acid or LSD is probably the most well-known and notorious hallucinogenic drug. Other well-known hallucinogens include psilocybin, which occurs naturally in certain wild mushrooms, commonly known as magic mushrooms or shrooms, and mescaline, which is found in peyote cactus in Mexico and the Southwestern United States.

Ecstasy is less hallucinogenic and more stimulating, which means more alertness than LSD or magical mushrooms. It is sometimes classified as a stimulant rather than a hallucinogen, and sometimes as an entactogen.

Less well-known neurotransmitter-like psychedelic drugs include Ololiuqui (found in the morning glory flower seeds).

Hallucinogens are a class of drugs that cause deep distortions in the perceptions of a person's reality, otherwise known as hallucinations. When users may see images under the influence of hallucinogens, hear sounds or experience sensations that appear to be real but are not.

Nearly all hallucinogens have nitrogen content and are known as alkaloids. Many hallucinogens have similar chemical structures to those of naturally occurring neurotransmitters (acetylcholine, serotonin, or catecholamine).

The most ordinarily abused hallucinogens are:

- LSD
- Mescaline
- Psilocybin
- PCP
- DMT
- Ayahuasca

Hallucinogens can be man-made, or they can emerge out of plants or mushrooms or concentrates from plants and mushrooms. For the most part, they are partitioned into two types: classic hallucinogens (LSD) or dissociative drugs (PCP). Either type of hallucinogen can cause users to have fast, serious enthusiastic swings.

Regular Hallucinogens

A portion of the more typical hallucinogens include:

LSD

D-lysergic corrosive diethylamide (LSD) is a manmade chemical made from ergot, an organism that develops on specific grains. It is presumably the most remarkable hallucinogen accessible, creating mental trips, changes in the way reality is seen, and adjusted moods.

It comes as a white powder or clear fluid and has no shading or smell. It can come in containers, however, frequently goes ahead little squares of blotter paper or gelatin that users place on the tongue or swallow to take a "trip."

Mescaline

A characteristic substance found as the fundamental fixing in the peyote cactus. The highest point of the gutless peyote cactus plants has plate molded "buttons" that contain mescaline.

The buttons are dried out and afterward either bit or absorbed fluid to produce an inebriating drink. Mescaline can likewise be made through chemical synthesis.

Psilocybin

A characteristic substance that is found in hallucinogenic mushrooms that contain psilocybin and psilocin.

In enormous enough dosages, psilocybin can produce effects fundamentally the same as the ground-breaking hallucinogen LSD. "Shrooms" as they are once in a while called can be used either new or dried. They are typically eaten, blended in with nourishment, or brewed like tea for drinking.

PCP

PCP is a hazardous manmade substance that was initially evolved as a sedative yet was ended for human use in 1965 because of symptoms. It is currently an illicit street drug sold as a white powder or in fluid structure. It tends to be grunted, infused, smoked, or gulped.

It produces pipedreams and "out-of-body" sensations. Utilization, particularly in huge dosages, can be dangerous and lead to genuine psychological well-being problems.

DMT

Dimethyltryptamine, otherwise called Dimitri, is a characteristic chemical found in some Amazonian plant species, however it can likewise be chemically synthesized. It normally comes as a white, crystalline powder that is disintegrated or smoked in a funnel or bong.

Ayahuasca

Here and there called hoasca, aya, and yage, ayahuasca is brewed from plants containing DMT alongside an Amazonian vine that forestalls the typical breakdown of DMT in the stomach related system. It is generally devoured like tea.

Researchers don't know precisely how hallucinogens and dissociative drugs produce their effects on the user. However, classic hallucinogens are thought to influence neural circuits in the brain including the synapse serotonin, and dissociative drugs cause their effects by basically disturbing the activities of the brain's glutamate system.

The locales of the brain that are influenced by hallucinogens control mood, tangible discernment, rest, hunger, body temperature, sexual behavior, and muscle control.

The pharmacology of psilocybin

Psilocybin-containing mushrooms are one of the major hallucinogenic drugs of abuse today. These mushroom species are distributed worldwide, and their abuse potential produces incompletely destructive effects in a developing populace of psychedelic drug users. No physical harm however numerous mental entanglements have been accounted for worldwide. Late research has been accounted for on the treatment of impulsive issue in humans with psilocybin; in this manner, it is critical to know the fundamental pharmacological data about psilocybin. Regardless of the way that unadulterated manufactured psilocybin (Indocybin® Sandoz) was used and showcased for experimental and psychotherapeutic purposes during the 1960s, as of not long ago just restricted pharmacological data were accessible. As of late some experimental psychophysiological considers were acted in which human pharmacokinetic and pharmacodynamic data of psilocybin were investigated further because of the generally scattered material about the pharmacological properties of psilocybin, old and new data are looked into here. It ought to be noticed that portrayal of the complex psychopathological phenomenainudced isn't in the focal point of this survey.

Pharmacology of Psilocybin (4-phosphoryloxy-N, N-dimethyltryptamine) is a subbed Indole alkylamine and has a place with the gathering of hallucinogenic tryptamines. Psilocybin was separated from Central American mushrooms (Psilocybe mexicana) by the prestigious Swiss physicist Albert

Hofmann in 1957, and in 1958 was produced artificially just because psilocybin was found to produce a well-controllable modified condition of cognizance. This state is set apart by incitement of effect, upgraded capacity for thoughtfulness and adjusted mental working toward Freudian essential procedures, referred to in any case as hypnagogic experience and dreams. Especially important are perceptual changes, for example, fantasies, synesthesia, affective activation, and modifications of thought and time sense. The effects last from 3 to 6 hours. After broad tests in creatures and humans, psilocybin was distributed worldwide under the name Indocybin® (Sandoz) as a short-acting and progressively perfect substance (than, for instance, LSD) to help psychotherapeutic procedures. Experimental and restorative use was broad and without entanglements.

Somatic effects

Cerletti reported an LD50 for mice with a 280 mg / kg intravenous application that could imply an LD50 of some grams of psilocybin in humans. In some in vitro experiments psilocybin showed no specific effects on isolated organs (intestines, heart) of guinea pigs and rats, except for an inhibitory effect on the neurotransmitter serotonin. Characteristic autonomic effects of the neurovegetative system notable to the entire animal (mice, rats, rabbits, cats and dogs) at 10 mg / kg s.c. doses. Included: mydriasis, piloting, heart and breathing irregularities, and discrete hyperglycemic and hypertonic effects. Cerletti interpreted these effects as an exciting syndrome caused by central sympathetic system stimulation. Motor activity was reduced as opposed to an autonomic excitatory syndrome. Experiments with Rhesus monkeys (2–4 mg / kg i. p.) verified the above improvements in physiological parameters and a central excitatory syndrome. The EEG has shown a disappearance of alpha activity and an increase of beta activity in the neo-cortex after 20–40 minutes. In two early non-blind studies in healthy volunteers (n= 12, 0.12–0.15 mg / kg p.o.), (n= 22, 10 mg p.o.), the EEG showed variations in the potential evoked by the visual and decrease in alpha and theta. Electroretinogram did not change. The somatic effects in humans were first investigated in healthy volunteers by Quetinin, a non-blind study (n= 29, 8–12 mg p.o., i.m.). Table 1 lists the physiological changes which have been noted regularly. Another early non-blind study (n= 16, 0.11 mg / kg p.o.) confirmed these effects qualitatively. Discrete changes in RR and pulse were also confirmed in a recent double-blind placebo-controlled study (n= 8, 0.2 mg / kg p.o.), as shown in Table 2.9 The effects described were barely noticeable and should be interpreted as secondary pharmacological effects, induced primarily by sympathomimetic e Hollister et al. found no significant aberrations of the aforementioned parameters in one subject following administration of psilocybin for 21 consecutive days with increased dosages (1.5 mg increased to 25 mg p.o. in three doses per day). Electrolyte levels, measures of liver toxicity and blood sugar levels remained unchanged.

Chapter 4

The Fungal Life Cycle

To get a good sense of exactly what the fungi are, it helps to understand what they're doing for a living, how they're getting around and what kind of love they're leading. A good way to get a handle on this is to trace the cycle of fungal life, the journey from birth to death, with each successive generation repeated endlessly. Knowing the life cycles of organisms is an ideal way to sort out what is unique to each, as no two species do the same. Sexual reproduction is a recombination of the genetic material to form a new one from two parent individuals.

The genetic material that each parent donates is known as a gamete. The fungal gametes are called spores. A spore is a compact, protected cell, able to stay alive but dormant for long periods of time until it finds an appropriate home. All the fungi that we will address in this book are known as Basidiomycetes because they grow their spores on basidia, tiny baseball-bat-shaped protuberances lining their gills, the blade-like structures arranged in a circular pattern on the underside of the cap, or pileus. The pileus, known to mycologists as a stipe, is held aloft on the end of a cylindrical stem.

Spore Discharge

Let's come back to our cow patty and its solitary mushroom. Zoom in closer: deep in darkness, millions of small, baseball-bat-shaped basidia stick out from the flat faces of the gills lining the underside of the parasol, and four ovoid, purple-black spores stand at the wide end of each basidium. At the outer end of the basidium, known as a sterigmata, each spore is perched like a top upon a tiny horn-shaped protuberance. Thanks to the wonders of evaporative cooling taking place on the sun-beaten upper face of the cap, the air around the gills is moist and much cooler than that around the mushroom.

Water condenses around the spore and its tiny stand as the air cools, and a droplet begins to form at the place they join in. The droplet grows until it can no longer bear its own structure, its surface tension breaks, and the droplet water spreads over the spore's body. The action's force pushes the spore towards the sterigma.

Being somewhat elastic, the stigma collapses slightly below the spore's weight, only to push back with an equal and opposite force and catapult the spore from its perch into the open space beyond the gills ' face. The amount of force is calculated precisely to hurtle the spore far enough to clear the surface of its own gill, but not so far that it smacks into the one facing. Instead, it succumbs to gravity and is pulled straight down and out under the mushroom's bottom face, where, with a little bit of luck, it will be carried away by a breeze of wind along with millions of its siblings. When the wind subsides in our field, two spores from our mushroom have settled on a patch of grass, where they are now patiently waiting for something or someone to bring them closer together.

Fungal Growth

Now picture a cow, perhaps the one who made that same cow patty from at chapter beginning. The cow mumbles on the grass in our field, because that's what cows like to do, and sooner or later she eats the grass blades on which our solitary spores sit, mumming them down with her lunch. Swallowed with the grass too, they are washed through her digestive tract only to emerge at the other end sometime later. Fortunately, through the guts of the cow, the spores are robust and well-armed, and do not experience any ill effects from their wildlife. Better still, they find themselves smacked in the middle of a mound of their food for their troubles: cow poop. Shortly afterwards, each of our spores germinates, splitting its cells into the delectable, nutrient-rich materials in the cow patty and slowly growing out.

Growing fungi consist of hyphae networks: tubular, filamentous cells which expand and divide at their forward tips, occasionally branching to create fork-or tan-like structures. Masses of hyphae are collectively known as the fungal mycelium. To the naked eye, fungal mycelium often appears on the surface of the food source (or substratum) as white, fuzzy or hair-like growth, as you may see at the underside of an upturned log.

Many fungi spend most of their days as an undifferentiated mycelium, creating only rarely specialized, complex structures such as chestnuts. Hyphal growth is also invasive, meaning it occurs throughout the substratum, and often within. Digestive enzymes secreted from the tips of the advancing mycelium turn the substrate into simpler organic molecules, to be absorbed or swallowed up by the mycelium as it marches. Fungi do their digestion outdoors, in effect. While we tend to process our meals inside our own privacy, fungi prefer eating out. All the fungi we discuss in this book are saprophytes, or saprobes, which means that they derive their nutrition from non-living organic matter, dead or decaying plants in this case. This contrasts with parasitic fungi that colonize and digest living organisms, often ending up killing their host, and mycorrhizal fungi that live in a symbiotic relationship with their host plants.

Herbal Ally - Mysterious Mushrooms

As summer evenings extend into fall, the timberlands of the Catskill Mountains in upstate New York load up with otherworldly, magical, medicinal mushrooms. "Toadstool" is a curious name for the numerous mushrooms that spring forward between downpours, while "fungi" is the more specialized term. Fungi are plants, however plants without blossoms or roots or chlorophyll (which makes plants green). Peculiar shapes (some explicitly intriguing), the ability to develop (and gleam) in obscurity, and psychedelic hues make mushrooms a conspicuous expansion to any witch's stew. However, you will need some different motivations to make mushrooms a steady piece of your eating regimen. Is outmaneuvering cancer a sufficient explanation?

It's valid. Every single palatable parasite - including those conventional white catch mushrooms sold in supermarkets - are fit for forestalling and turning around cancerous cell changes. We aren't actually certain why. Maybe this is because fungi search out, concentrate, and share with us the follow minerals we have to manufacture ground-breaking, healthy invulnerable systems. Or on the other hand maybe this is because of their abundance of polysaccharides - fascinating complex sugars that have all the earmarks of being all round health-advertisers. It could be because mushrooms are astounding wellsprings of protein and B nutrients with barely any calories and no sodium. Or then again, we could single out the anti-cancer, anti-tumor, and anti-bacterial mixes found in the stalk, tops, gills, and even the underground structures (mycelia) of each eatable mushroom.

Make certain to cook your mushrooms however; abstain from eating them crude. Researchers at the University of Nebraska Medical School found that mice who ate boundless measures of crude mushrooms (Agaricusbisporus) created, throughout their lifetimes, essentially more dangerous tumors than a control gathering.

Wherever I go in August and September - in the case of strolling shoeless on lively green greeneries or venturing softly over the profoundly scented fallen pine and hemlock needles; in the case of climbing rough outcrops trimmed with ferny hairs or evading swamps murmuring with mosquitoes; in the case of following the sloppy bank of a wandering stream or adjusting on old stone dividers breathing in the fragrance of noble decay - I am vigilant for my fungi companions.

My woods are particularly liberal to me with chanterelles, wonderful cornucopia-molded mushrooms with a delightful taste. I find both the flavorful minimal dark ones - tongue in cheek known as "trumpet of death" because of their scary hue - and the exceptionally scrumptious and a lot of bigger orange ones. Some of the time we get back bare from our mushroom's strolls - in the event that we find a bigger number of mushrooms than we have packs for, we need to use our shirts and jeans as bearers to help pull supper home.

The splendid orange tops and sulfur yellow undersides of sulfur rack mushrooms (Polyporussulphuroides) are anything but difficult to spot in the pre-fall woodland. Becoming just on as of late dead oaks, these covering racks make an incredible tasting resistant improving expansion to supper. I have harvested the "chicken of the woods" in oak backwoods around the globe. In the Czech Republic, I considered to be enormous model as we drove a nation path. Halting, I found a bit of it had been harvested. I took just a share, being mindful so as to leave parts for other mushroom darlings who may descend the path after me.

You don't need to live in the woods and find your own mushrooms to make the most of their health-giving advantages. You can buy them: new or dried for use in cooking and medicine; and tinctured or powdered too. Search for chanterelles, cepes, enoki, clam mushrooms, portobellos, maitake, reishii, shiitake, chaga, and numerous other fascinating and medicinal mushrooms in health nourishment stores, supermarkets, claim to fame stores, and Oriental markets.

Maitake (Grifoliafrondosa) is more effective than some other fungi at any point tried at restraining tumor development. It is effective when taken orally, regardless of whether by guinea pigs or humans dealing with cancer. The fruiting body of the maitake looks like the tail plumes of a little dark colored chicken, thus its famous name: "Hen of the Woods". In the event that you buy maitake in pill structure, make certain to get the fruiting body, not the mycelium.

Reishii (Ganodermalucidum) is one of the most regarded safe tonics in the world. Reishii is adaptogenic, rejuvenating, and regenerative, particularly to the liver. Indeed, even intermittent use fabricates ground-breaking invulnerability and diminishes the danger of cancer. In clinical examinations, use of reishii expanded T-cell and alpha interferon creation, shrank and killed tumors, and improved the personal satisfaction for terminal patients. Reishii and shiitake are incredible accomplices, the effects of one upgrading the effects of the other. Reishii is best taken as a tincture, 20-40 drops, and multiple times every day.

Shiitake (Lentinusedodes) is exceptionally medicinal and tastes adequate to eat in quantity. I go to an oriental market and buy the big, big, big sack of dried shiitake mushrooms for a small amount of what I would pay for them in a health nourishment store. To use, I just rehydrate them by pouring bubbling water over them or by dropping pieces into soups. The individuals who make shiitake a customary piece of their weight control plans increment their creation of cancer-battling alpha interferon, decrease irritation all through their bodies, delay their lives, and improve their ability to produce and use nutrient D.

Chaga (Inonotus obliquus) is a somewhat appalling and strongly hard fungi found on birch trees. Baba Yaga and other Russian cultivators favor it as an invulnerable nourisher, cancer preventive, and a guide to those dealing with melanomas.

Mushrooms are not only for nourishment and medicine; they are famous for their ability to change our impression of reality. Psychoactive psilocybin mushrooms were used by the popular shaman/healer Maria Sabina in Mexico. The red-topped mushroom with white specks normally attracted by the witch's house is the brain adjusting Amanita muscaria, in some cases called sustenance, and generally used in Siberian shamanic customs.

Regardless of whether you use fungi to make a mushroom soup or as a solution for somebody dealing with cancer, whether you work them up in a witch's cauldron of spiraling power or sew them into a soul pack, mushrooms offer enchantment and secret, great health and encouragement.

Types of Psilocybin Mushrooms

Various types of psilocybin mushrooms are found on pretty much every landmass. They are otherwise called psychedelic or enchantment mushrooms because of the psychoactive substances they contain. These chemicals are called psilocybin, psilocin, and baeocystin, and they are what give the mushrooms their hallucinogenic symptoms.

However, when we talk about psilocybin mushrooms, there are not only a couple of various types to choose from. In fact, there are in excess of 180 distinct species of psilocybin mushrooms developing in nature. Also, these various types fall into a couple of various class classifications.

Various Types of Psilocybin Mushrooms

A large portion of the psilocybin mushrooms are found in the Psilocybe family. In fact, this one has in any event 126 unique species of psilocybin mushrooms to choose from, all shifting in size, shape, coloring, and intensity. These various species are found everywhere throughout the world, so regardless of where you will be, you can get your hands on at any rate one type of Psilocybe mushroom.

However, there other distinctive psilocybin mushroom genera out there which despite everything contain the psychedelic chemicals. These ones don't have the same number of various species varieties as the Psilocybe mushrooms; however, they are as yet important. These genera include:

- Conocybe
- Copelandia
- Galerina
- Gymnopilus
- Inocybe
- Mycena
- Panaeolus
- Pholiotina
- Pluteus

Presently, it ought to be noticed that not the entirety of the various species in every one of the genera recorded above are psilocybin mushrooms. For example, the vast majority of the species in the Inocybe variety are noxious, making it somewhat troublesome — and conceivably risky — to find the psychedelic ones.

Psilocybin Mushrooms Representative Species

If you've chosen to proceed to look at a couple of the mushrooms in your area, there are a couple of species that share comparable highlights, for example, dull spores and gills. What's more, huge numbers of them are found in similar areas of the world, making them a lot simpler to find. These mushrooms are known as the psilocybin mushrooms delegate species, because of the likenesses between them.

Psilocybecubensis

This is the most well-known species around. Additionally called "shapes" or "shrooms," it very well may be found developing on dairy animal's compost along the Gulf Coast in the U.S. yet, develops in Mexico, Central America, South America, and the West Indies also. It can likewise be found in parts of Asia and Australia.

Young mushrooms begin with bended tops, yet they smooth out as the mushroom ages. They develop somewhere in the range of 2-8 cm in diameter. The coloring is rosy brown from the start however helps to a brilliant brown. The spore prints of these mushrooms are a dim purple brown.

Psilocybecyanescens

This one is designated "wavy tops" because of the unmistakable waves that structure right now the mushroom ages. Its coloring is pale and yellowish, which is uncommon among these mushrooms. However, its blackish-brown spores are very normal in the class.

These mushrooms develop on wood chips, favoring areas wealthy in lignin. They can be found in the Pacific Northwest areas of the U.S., just as in parts of Europe and New Zealand.

Psilocybemexicana

Generally, these were used by the Aztecs and Mayans for strict and profound functions for a huge number of years. They are known for their little 2-3 cm tops that are brown or beige when young yet help to a straw shading after some time. They may even have blue or green tones to them at times. These ones additionally have the dull spore prints and the mushroom even turns blue when wounded.

Psilocybesemilanceata

Known as "Freedom Caps," these basic mushrooms develop in the knolls and fields of North America and Europe; however, they lean toward the sheep munching grounds over the steers areas. One of the strongest mushrooms around, these ones have tops going from 5-25 mm in diameter. These tops roll internal when young yet unroll and may even twist up as the mushroom ages. Like the other agent species, this one has a brown or purple spore print.

In the event that you are a novice to the world of psilocybin mushrooms, the normal highlights make these ones simple to recognize. However, you ought to never ingest a mushroom in the event that you don't know what kind it is. Do a legitimate spore print to be certain you have the correct one, or you may endure some quite awful results.

Chapter 5

How to Grow Mushrooms - Learn About Growing Mushrooms

Not many people realize that it is actually very easy to cultivate mushrooms yourself at home, instead choosing to spend their money on cheaply imported mushroom species from foreign countries where they are cultivated in bulk at their local supermarket. The shop variety doesn't have much of a shelf life and the mushrooms don't really like being packed in plastic so learning to grow mushrooms at home will not only give you fresher longer-lasting mushrooms but they will also most likely taste stronger and more mushrooms as the shop varieties tend to have a more watered-down flavor.

Another advantage of cultivating mushrooms yourself is that you're not limited to the variety shown in the shops-which usually consists of mushroom buttons, Shiitake, Oyster and Portobello. Although you see Oyster mushrooms as the easiest type of mushroom to grow, you may want to try to grow something that most shops will never sell. The Lions Mane mushroom is a bit harder to grow and yet has a very similar taste to that of lobster and it is very expensive to buy from specialist retailers.

You'll need to decide on a variety to be able to grow your own mushrooms first. There are hundreds of edible mushrooms that can be grown either inside your house or outside, most growers settle for the oyster mushroom to start with because of the simplicity of growing it (Oyster, or Pleutorus Ostreateus has very vigorous growth and so is very likely to grow under the right conditions).

Once you have decided to grow a type of mushroom you will need to find the unique growing criteria, as all mushrooms have their own growing parameters. You can use either a wood-based substratum (paper, carton etc.) with the Oyster mushroom or you can grow it on straw. These are the most commonly used substrates, as they provide the highest yield.

The next thing you need is the spawning mushroom. It's easiest to buy your spawn from a shop-which is probably easiest done online, as most garden centers only sell complete mushroom growing kits, while the spawn is a little more specialist on its own. There are many websites that sell spawn and a bag that will provide you with lots of mushrooms will only cost you a few pounds (it's also much better to grow your own mushrooms then buy them from a store).

You need to pasteurize the straw or paper-based product with the oyster mushrooms which kills many of the bacteria present, giving the mushroom a head-start when growing. This can be done by submerging the straw / paper in some hot water, keeping it for about 1 hour at around 60 degrees C. Drain the substrate when this has been finished, and allow it to cool before putting it into a plastic bag. Place a handful of straw / paper in the bag and sprinkle spawn on top, then proceed until the bag is full. Tie the bag with a metal tie and pierce holes over the bag, allowing air to help the mycelium grow and allowing mushrooms to grow later. Keep it in a warm room for about 2 weeks until the bag colonizes fully (turns white, from the mycelium growing). An ideal place is an airing dresser or boiler room).

When the bag is fully colonized it will be ready for fruit- within a few days mushrooms should begin to appear. You need to switch the bag to a warmer, damper region where the humidity levels are around 90 percent or higher to help it get fruit. Oyster mushrooms like to be in fairly cool conditions so it's probably best to put them outside. They will start forming (pin) from previously poked holes in the jar, due to the mushrooms that liked the air given. When this happens, cut the bag carefully and peel it back a bit, allowing the mushrooms to grow to large sizes with the air and space required. When the Oyster mushrooms look good size and unfurl just before the caps release their spores, pull them gently and twist them to harvest them at their stems. With a knife, cut the end part of the stem and they'll be ready to eat!

Where Do 'Shrooms Grow?

While you are eating your mushrooms, ever ponder where do these little children grow? Ever wonder how could they occur?

All things considered, first off, mushrooms, genuine, they grow over the ground, well the greater part of them. In any case, unlike plants that need daylight and water to thrive, mushrooms scarcely need these two. Also, absolutely never feel that you are going to plant mushrooms utilizing some mushroom seeds!

As much the same number of adoration mushrooms, they have a place with a similar arrangement as those fungi that unleash ruin on the skin. However, mind you, the ones you eat don't influence you except if you are susceptible to them. We should get down to the rudiments: mushrooms are fungi. Indeed, they are. However, they are far separated from the one you see on the restroom floor. The ones individuals eat are in reality only a piece of the eatable assortment. Be it clam, shitake or piece, what individuals have been eating up is really the conceptive piece of the mushroom. Maybe this may be the motivation behind why mushrooms have been thought of as a Spanish fly. Since you have known and taken care of business on mushroom data, knowing where this grow is additionally important.

Like numerous things right now, don't simply pop anyplace. It might look that way, yet it is really the opposite. Indeed, even in their indigenous habitat, mushrooms have a few requirements as well. So, in case you wish to cultivate mushrooms, you have to mimic these requirements to create better looking and better tasting mushrooms. Notwithstanding that, you have to have a procedure, so you don't depend on chance when you need to cultivate mushrooms professionally or even similarly as a leisure activity.

Where do mushrooms grow?

Think moist, spoiled logs. These are the areas generally helpful for mushroom growth in nature. The best place for mushrooms to thrive is in a dim place, with dampness, and there is a nourishment source. Presently, you may think about what kind of nourishment mushrooms need-the carbohydrates-found in spoiling grass and wood. That is the place they get their sustenance.

How?

It is in the mycelium. Think about the mycelium as the base of the mushrooms. The mycelium holds fast to the substrate, right now, decaying wood. The better the hyphae or the string like part adheres to the wood, the all the more tasting the mushroom becomes. The mycelium is likewise important in shipping the supplements to the mushroom. When you see these minor globs called pins, this implies the correct kind of blend has been accomplished. These "pins" will turn into the mushrooms we eat once it gets develop.

It is additionally important to observe the various types of substrate to use for development of various types of mushroom. For example, shitakes thrive best on logs and wooden chips. Then again, shellfish mushrooms favor clean straws. Isn't it great that mushroom development just expects you to spend close to nothing? You basically simply need to request some waste wood chips and use these to begin you claim mushroom garden at home.

Simple Tips on How to Grow Mushrooms

Would you like to figure out how to grow mushrooms? There are a wide range of mushroom growing packs available that can kick you off, however there are a couple of insider facts that the units don't let you know. Other than the mushroom growing pack (or mushroom spores), you'll need the accompanying household things:

- electric fan
- spray mist bottle
- cooking oil spray

Tip #1:

Set up the mushroom pack in a place where the temperature is steady. Depending on where you live and what your normal day by day temperature is, you might need to explore different avenues regarding better places to grow your mushrooms.

Tip #2:

Don't put your mushroom confine legitimately front of a window. Give aberrant light, however not immediate sunlight. All the more light can cause certain mushroom tops to turn dull brown.

Tip #3:

Mist the mushroom block every day with a spray bottle. Consistent stickiness is important for the mushrooms to create and grow. In the event that you live in a dry atmosphere, you may need to mist all the more regularly. In the event that your atmosphere is as of now moist, you won't need to spray as frequently.

Tip #4:

Give air flow. Mushrooms need a great deal of air to forestall carbon dioxide develop. An excess of carbon dioxide will make your mushroom creation stop don't as well, attempt to grow mushrooms in a little storage room or an encased space.

Tip # 5:

At the point when the cover that appends the top to the stem starts to tear, it's a great opportunity to collect - ordinarily after around about fourteen days in the light. Depending on your mushrooms, it might be the point at which the mushrooms are the size of a marble or the size of an orange. Turn the block day by day to check for harvestable mushrooms that might be hanging out. Tenderly turn and pull mushrooms from the block. Halfway stems left on the block will spoil, so don't cut them.

Tip # 6:

Problems with insects? Shield your mushrooms from insects by spraying the folds of the growing box with cooking oil spray. The oil will trap and execute the insects before they arrive at your mushrooms.

Chapter 6

Growing Mushrooms Indoors

Did you look for an alternate way to grow some kind of food indoors during another time than your usual gardening season? Should you live in an extremely low area where your daily temperatures drop? Looking for an alternative way to raise the equivalent amount of food you'd have in a tiny garden patch? If this is an issue for you then maybe this article would benefit you somewhat.

As with any type of plant, you must understand that according to the inverse square law, the light intensity of your growing area descends. What this means is that a light half the distance from your plant would give you four times the light energy that gets to the plant. You should always look for plants in this respect which you can effectively position closer to the lights you have mounted. Examples of that would have been sprouts. Sprouts grow easily and take up very little space. They generally do very well with an indoor environment and offer a welcome addition to your current diet.

The one thing you need to keep in mind is the amount of money you'll be spending on electricity to power your growth lights. Even in those areas where you can normally grow vegetables outdoors it never hurts during the spring months to start your plants inside.

Raising some mushrooms would be one excellent solution. Growing mushrooms can be achieved any time of the year in any climate. They also provide a good supplement to your usual diet.

Mushrooms are perfect for improving your cooking flavor, and you are provided with many varieties to choose from. You don't need a formal garden to grow then and they can easily be raised in dark crawl spaces beneath your home because they are a fungus. Mushrooms are one of the few plants that grow without the chlorophyll benefit. This means the plant must receive all of its nutrition from the material upon which it grows. A mix of pulverized corn cobs or straw with nitrogen supplements and added gypsum is one of the best materials for growing your mushrooms in. If you feel like being a do it yourself then use a little rice flour and vermiculite to easily create your own medium. You just need to spread it out over your holding bin.

There are many retailers online that can provide you with mushroom kits that are complete with spores and all the supplies you need to grow them in the comforts of your home. A choice of the ever-popular Portabella, Crimini, Beech, Enoki, Shiitake or a host of other great mushrooms is presented when selecting your variety to grow. Since each one will have its own cultural requirements, you should carefully read the enclosed instructions.

Usually the mushroom kits range in price from $25 and up depending on how you plan to grow it. These little gems can even be grown using sterile pots. Fill each jar with your chosen medium and distribute the spores over it. You can install a sort of dome housing on the jar to regulate the amount of moisture and the temperature.

Mushroom Grow Box for Small Spaces

Some mushrooms grow only in the tiny space that our naked eyes cannot see. Others are also cultivated to cultivate different kinds of mushrooms in a log or even in boxes, since they don't have enough space inside their homes, or their area is not suitable for cultivating this kind. Some others also believe that mushrooms grown in a box are grown efficiently and productively because the owner gives them a lot of attention.

Another most common thing about the whole mushroom grow box is its size which fits all spaces. You can always have the mushroom cultivated inside your home during winter months. That, apart from that, is so true in all other areas of your home where you can see its natural growth in the very little space provided. In some cases, mushrooms are already supplied on the box, so you only need to check the temperature for proper growth on the box itself. Magic mushrooms are mostly planted on these boxes because they are less likely to be small than other types. Besides that, the mushroom grow box has its own specific size that is suitable for all styles. Few interesting facts are that it can grow easily within weeks and can collect from 250 to 350 pieces of magic mushroom (only for this type). Check also for the pH level of the soil, so that on boxes mushrooms grow independently. Somehow, the box casing is already installed in such a way that soil can allow its moist impact to turn more mushrooms on the grow box. A tip for you: you can also place the growing box in your refrigerator so that the soil's humidity increases its natural efficiency and your mushrooms can be cultivated efficiently.

Mushroom grow box is not only intended for small spaces but also for large areas. It depends only on the owner's perception of the commodity and mushroom which he wants to cultivate. On the other hand, the box should be made and neatly covered to avoid spreading other not so good fungi which will affect its growth. The mushroom grow box is made for easy placement all over the place. You need to be more knowledgeable about this quite obviously so that growing mushrooms won't be a waste on your part.

Mushroom Compost - Organic Vegetable Garden Benefits

Spent mushroom compost, likewise, known as "spent mushroom substrate" or "mushroom soil," is quickly developing in fame for natural soil altering. Harvests thrive with 7 natural vegetable garden benefits of mushroom compost. For the most part containing coconut hulls, roughage, corn cobs, cottonseed meal, poultry manure and straw horse bedding, the unadulterated compost is dim, rich and scentless.

1) Completely reused

This compost is the disposed of after mushrooms have grown in it. New compost must be used once to grow mushrooms, so the used or spent compost must be discarded. One excellent way to reuse these "scraps" is to sustain your vegetable garden. Thought about a sustainable option in contrast to peat moss, reused compost can likewise help spare the peat lowlands' fragile natural parity.

2) Adds natural issue to the soil

Much the same as customary natural garden compost, microbial activity is created as it separates, creating humus. Excellent at separating clay soil, revise liberally in your soil to create a rich loamy texture. Recollect that all organics keep on separating. Following a couple of months, you may need to add a top layer to container plants. A 3 to 6-inch open air application is relied upon to last 2 to 5 years.

3) Drought safe

Compost monitors dampness to plants by expanding the ability to hold water, while circulating air through the soil simultaneously. The parasitic activity of past mushroom growing creates a clammy hindrance against dry season and burning heat. This is excellent for vegetable gardens by improving soil structure and sparing water costs, particular in dry zones.

4) Controls Garden Pests

Mushroom compost is natural issue that creates great microbial activity. Helpful microorganisms thusly support advantageous insects, earth worm activity and debilitate sicknesses. All these regular controls assist gardeners with evading the use of possibly hazardous garden chemicals that can hurt our earth and threaten our family and pet health.

5) Fast growing plants and vegetables

Research shows gainful organism or mycorrhizae work with plants to produce synergistic vitality that outcomes in quick growth. Since spent mushroom compost used to host mushrooms, it is brimming with this great parasite and reports flourish about awesome plant growth. Normally low in nitrogen, mushroom compost doesn't energize over verdant growth, making it perfect for flower bearing plants like vegetables.

6) Weed free

Mushrooms must be grown in medium that has been disinfected and composted, so the left-over compost is weed and plant pathogen free. This makes flawless mulch for vegetable and flower gardens, trees, bushes and top dressings for existing yards. With this compost you can be sure you are not acquiring undesirable weed seeds to rival your plants.

7) Pleasant smelling

Appropriately made and put away, this compost doesn't smell horrible. In fact, it has a practically sweet smell when new. Indeed, even that scent rapidly disseminates once put in the ground. A reviving alleviation for gardeners wherever who might be used to bovine or poultry manures as natural compost. Never again will your neighbors shoot you filthy searches for growing natural. Whenever spent mushroom compost has a foul scent, don't use it except if you re-compost.

How to Plant Mushrooms - Grow Your Own Oyster Mushrooms Indoors

Oyster mushrooms are one of the easiest mushroom varieties to grow and learning how to plant mushrooms will offer you nearly unlimited supply of the mushrooms at your dining table. Although oyster mushrooms grow in woods, you can use other growing media to raise them. Think of straw and sawdust, they're easier to collect than logs.

Oyster mushroom resembles oysters and has a rich history of gastronomy and medicine to boast. Starting about three thousand years ago, Chinese medicine uses oyster mushrooms as a tonic to strengthen the immune system. It has ergothioneine, an exceptional antioxidant able to protect the cell. Even when the oyster mushrooms are cooked, the level of antioxidants remains the same. It has been proven that the mushrooms have anti-bacterial properties too. Oyster mushrooms have significant potassium, iron, zinc, vitamin C, calcium, niacin, phosphorus, B1 and B2 vitamins, and folic acid content. The study revealed eating oyster mushrooms contributes to the dietary requirements suggested.

Commercially prepared mushrooms contain pesticides and other chemicals to make them presentable and for longer shelf-life. While mushrooms may make a considerable contribution to making you safe, the presence of harmful chemicals in them can shorten your life. The solution, right? Learn how to plant mushrooms and enjoy their many great benefits.

Preparations for your Search on How to Plant Mushrooms

In order to fill them in, you'll need two small cardboard boxes or milk cartons; two cups of coffee grounds or whole grain flour; oyster mushrooms spawn. If sawdust is not available or if you find it difficult to collect sawdust, then straw can always be used as a replacement (although sawdust is much better).

If you want to start with a kit, but if you want to start from scratch, then oyster mushrooms can give you a great margin over other mushroom varieties to make a success of your effort. Oyster mushrooms have dozens of different varieties to choose from and you can check with your supplier for the best variety appropriate for your spot. Many oyster mushrooms thrive in areas ranging from 55 to 65 degrees Fahrenheit.

The Steps you need to follow in Learning How to Plant Mushrooms.

The steps to follow in how mushrooms can be planted are not complicated, in fact they are easy to understand and follow. It does not demand that you be a genius to grow these mushrooms.

You'll need to cut the boxes you'll use to even height or the same size. Punch several holes in the sides of the two boxes or cartons (small in sizes but not as small as a pin).

If you choose to use pre-inoculated sawdust with spawn, do not sterilize the sawdust as it kills the spawn. If you use fresh sawdust, then you may want to first sterilize it. The sawdust can be steamed, heated, or micro welled. The sawdust can be steamed or boiled for a few minutes, and you can turn off the heat and keep it covered after sterilization. Let it cool before proceeding to next step at room temperature. If you opt for a microwave, you'll need to get a microwave-safe bowl and add the sawdust to the flour or coffee grounds. Fill it with sufficient water until the mixture looks like a damp sponge. When the water starts boiling it is going to kill the organisms you want to eliminate. To finish all of your sawdust, you might need to repeat the process in microwave.

For wash the sawdust, use unchlorinated spray. Make sure it is absolutely humid. Mix softly in your spores.

Pack the damp sawdust firmly into the boxes or cardboard boxes and leave it in a basement, garage, dark cabinet, locker or basement. Plastic can be wrapped beneath the container and covered with plastic with some cooking oil sprayed onto them to trap insects if any.

Keep the sawdust damp with unchlorinated water and enjoy the fruits of your work in a few months. Be sure to twist the mushrooms gently when harvesting, to avoid breaking the stem.

Learning how to plant mushrooms can also be a fun family activity which will benefit everyone in the long run.

Chapter 7

The Magical Mushroom

Mycology, the investigation of mushrooms, is carrying new admirers to the 'fungus among us." Already being used for an assortment of clinical reasons far and wide, the modest toadstool might be pushed into the spotlight soon as a fruitful, elective treatment for some difficult irregular characteristics.

Mushrooms are esteemed by veggie lovers because of their high healthy benefit. They can produce nutrient D when presented to sunlight. Mushrooms contain B nutrients, nutrient C, potassium, phosphorus, calcium, sodium, and zinc.

Medicinal mushrooms have thousands of mixes and supplements that are health-fortifying. Eastern medicine, particularly customary Chinese practices, has used mushrooms for a considerable length of time. In the U.S., studies were led in the mid '60s for potential ways to tweak the safe system and to restrain cancerous tumor growth with separates.

Mushroom chasing is mainstream; however, it isn't protected. Some consumable mushrooms are practically indistinguishable from poison ones. It takes a specialist to differentiate. Likewise, mushrooms act like a wipe and effectively retain poisons from soil and air. In any case, mushrooms are effortlessly viewed as a 'health nourishment.'

Without the procedure of photosynthesis, a few mushrooms acquire supplements by separating natural issue or by taking care of from higher plants. Another segment assault living plants to expend them. Palatable and toxic assortments are found close to foundations of oak, pine and fir trees.

Mushrooms were used customarily by the locals of Mesoamerica for thousands of years. They were broadly devoured in strict services by societies all through the Americas. Cavern works of art in Spain delineate ritualized ingestion going back similar to 9000 years. Psilocybin use was stifled until Western psychiatry rediscovered it after World War II.

The dubious area of research is the use of psilocybin, a normally occurring chemical in specific mushrooms. Psilocybin has been demonstrated to be effective in treating dependence on liquor and cigarettes.

New studies show the hallucinogenic drug may soothe nervousness and gloom in some cancer patients. Mood raising effects that endured in any event half a month in the wake of expending the fungus were accounted for in certain studies.

While fungus has intrigued individuals for quite a long time, it might at last be coming into another time where it's mending forces and obscure characteristics are being found. The mushroom might just hold the way in to sometime in the past bolted puzzles and illnesses.

Medicinal use of mushrooms has been continuing for thousands of years all things considered; they are effective. It is the ideal opportunity for increasingly focused research investigating extra uses and powers of this fragile blessing from nature.

Return of the Magic Mushroom

Mushrooms, also called toadstools, are fleshy fungal bodies that grow on the soil or on a food source above ground. In a kingdom they are isolated from the plant world all of their own called Myceteae because they do not produce chlorophyll like green plants.

Certain mushrooms obtain nutrients without the photosynthesis process by breaking down organic matter or feeding from higher plants. Those are called the decomposers. Another field is targeting live plants to kill and eat them and is called parasites. Edible and poisonous forms are mycorrhizal and can be found on or around trees roots such as oaks, pines, and firs.

Mushrooms can do one of three things for humans—nourish, cure or poison. Few are polite. The oyster, morel and chanterelles are the three most popular edible versions of this' meat of the vegetable world'

They are widely used in Chinese, Korean, Japan and Indian cuisine. In fact, China is the largest producer in the world, cultivating more than half of all mushrooms consumed worldwide. Most of the edible variety has been grown commercially on farms in our supermarkets and includes shiitake, portobello and enoki.

Eastern medicine has used mushrooms for decades, particularly traditional Chinese practices. In the United States, early 1960s studies were conducted on possible ways to modulate the immune system and inhibit tumor growth with extracts used in cancer research.

The Mesoamerican natives also used mushrooms ritually for thousands of years. Called by the Aztecs ' the flesh of the gods, mushrooms were widely consumed by cultures across the Americas in religious ceremonies. In Spain and Algeria, cave paintings depict ritualized ingestion dating back as far as 9000 years. Questioned by Religious leaders on both sides of the Atlantic, psilocybin use was discouraged until it was rediscovered by Western medicine after World War II. A 1957 essay in Life Magazine titled "Seeking the Magic Mushroom" sparked America's curiosity. The following year, Albert Hoffman, a Swiss scientist, identified psilocybin and psilocin as the active compounds in the 'magic' mushrooms. That prompted the creation of the Harvard Psilocybin Project at Harvard University led by American psychologist Timothy Leary to study the effects of the compound on humans.

In the next quarter century, psilocybin and other hallucinogens such as LSD and mescaline were given to 40,000 patients. More than 1,000 investigative papers have been published. Once the government became aware of the increasing subculture available to the use, laws were enforced.

The Nixon administration started regulations which included the 1970 Controlled Substances Act. The law created five timetables under which drugs were to be listed in growing severity. Psilocybin, along with marijuana and MDMA, was placed in the most stringent schedule I. Each was defined as having "high potential for abuse, no currently appropriate therapeutic use, and a lack of agreed protection." This ended the study for almost 25 years until recently, when studies opened up for potential use in treating or resolving PTSD-post-traumatic stress disorder along with anxiety issues. As of June 2014, 32 human clinical trials registered with the US have studied whole mushrooms or extracts. National health institutes and their potential impacts on a number of diseases and conditions. Many diseases that are treated include cancer, glaucoma, immune function, and inflammatory bowel disease.

The controversial area of research is the use of psilocybin, a chemical which occurs naturally in some mushrooms. It continues to explore its ability to help people suffering from psychological disorders such as obsessive-compulsive disorder, PTSD, and anxiety. In some studies psilocybin has also been shown to be effective in the treatment of alcohol and cigarette addiction.

While fungus has been fascinating people for centuries, it may end up entering a new era in which its healing powers and unknown qualities are being discovered. The mushroom might very well hold the key to some mysteries and diseases that had been locked up long ago.

The Magical Maitake Mushroom

What a chestnut this is! Part of the mushroom family that has now been classified as medicinal mushrooms, the Maitake mushroom is all in its own class. If you wish, a champion of sorts. The Maitake mushrooms are brimming with nutrition, unlike the regular button cap mushrooms we are all familiar with. Providing a wealth of protein, B-Vitamins, Vitamin-C, Niacin, Potassium, Selenium and a wealth of fiber sources, you can't go wrong to add Miatake mushrooms to the dinner menu. Maitake mushrooms taste great, with a rich flavor and a meaty texture. A side dish sautéed to perfection with this spectacular mushroom is the perfect complement to almost any menu.

The Maitake mushroom has its origin in the Japanese mountains. They are easily identified with a firm yet supple base by their cluster of dark fronds, which turn slightly crumbly at the edges. It's these dark fronds that mimic a hen's tail feathers that give them their notorious nicknames, "hen of the woods" or "dancing butterfly." In temperate forests in North America, we can now find Maitake mushrooms growing on deciduous hardwoods. There are now many companies that specialize in Maitake mushroom cultivation under strict, controlled environments. Naturally this in an effort to preserve the inherent and rich nutritional qualities of this revered species of mushrooms.

Maitake mushrooms are quickly becoming popular for their medicinal properties which occur naturally. This species ' purported uses in other countries include tumor inhibition, high blood sugar treatment, high cholesterol, high blood pressure and stimulation of the immune system. Maitake's medicinally active ingredients are found in the fruit bodies and the mycelium. In other countries, as a result of medicinal uses, there are now US laboratories and specialty producers specializing in the cultivation of the active agents found in Maitake mushrooms for use in nutraceutics. Medicinal extracts of this remarkable mushroom species can now be found for sale in holistic health care offices and health food stores across the US.

The maitake mushroom contains high concentrations of Beta 1, 3-1, 6 Glucans, a specialized molecule. These complex molecular and naturally occurring compounds are thought to improve the immune system's ability to function at an optimal level. Research suggests that cells of the immune system, such as macrophages, T-cells, and interleukin-1 cells, appear to be activating and functioning more aggressively when specialized Maitake compounds are taken orally. Recent research has also suggested that naturally occurring plant chemicals independent of the Beta compounds may also have tumor-fighting effects.

While research on the magical mushroom known as the Maitake is still young, there is sufficient early evidence to imply that further research is warranted regarding inherent health benefits. Knowledge in Maitake mushrooms and other members of the entire family of medicinal mushrooms has increased. The curiosity in the entire medicinal mushroom family has undergone a marked increase in the US over the last two decades. According to Harriet Benfield, acupuncturist and author, "The movement began with healthy food in the late 1960s. Now it's health medicine." Although it would be safe to say a fairly recent introduction to the U.S. diet, the Maitake mushroom will prove a valuable addition to the daily diet both. The Maitake extracts that occur naturally can also serve a beneficial function as part of a supplement regime.

Mushroom Magic

Who might have thought that a few types of mushroom hold magic health benefits? Research directed by Research Associate

Professor Min Zhang, School of Population Health at the University of Western Australia on the beneficial outcomes of eating mushrooms for women in China, demonstrates that they do, The Agaricus group of mushrooms have an uncommon enchantment, which has to a great extent gone unnoticed, that may give us a healthy high.

Current Research

Joint research attempted by Zhang from The University of Western Australia and Zhejiang University in China, found that eating mushrooms and drinking green tea may secure against breast cancer. Zhang detailed that breast cancer was the most widely recognized type of cancer among women worldwide and that its rate was expanding in both created and creating nations. Strangely, the rate of cancer in China was four or multiple times lower than in created nations. The examination would have liked to appear if this could be because of the use of dried and crisp mushrooms and green leaf tea in the customary Chinese eating regimen. Mushrooms, mushroom concentrates and green tea had indicated anti-cancer-causing properties which were thought to animate resistant responsiveness against breast cancer.

The utilization of mushrooms and green tea by 2,000 women, matured from 20 to 87 in generally well-to-do southeast China, was observed. Half of the women were healthy, and the others had affirmed breast cancer. On talk with, it was found that crisp white catch mushrooms, Agaricusbisporus, and fragrant dried mushrooms, Lentinula edodes, were the most normally eaten species of mushroom. A portion of the women in the examination devoured neither mushrooms nor green tea while others appreciated both up to three times each day.

The consequences of the examination indicated that the blend of a dietary admission of mushrooms and green tea diminished breast cancer hazard with an extra decreased effect on the harm of cancer. Zhang inferred that, whenever affirmed reliably in other research, this reasonable dietary intercession may have potential ramifications for assurance against breast cancer advancement.

Dr. W. J. Sinden from University of Pennsylvania and Dr. E. D. Lambert from Lambert Laboratories were the first to exhibit their research results on the medicinal mixes of Agaricusblazei. They pulled in the consideration of the clinical network to this mushroom. Previous President Ronald Reagan used this mushroom to battle his skin cancer, which helped publicize Agaricusblazei.

How Do Mushrooms Help Fight Cancer?

The Agaricusblazei mushroom is made up of Beta-(1-3) - D-glucan, Beta-(1-4)- a - D-glucan& Beta - (1-6)- D-glucan. Known as Beta Glucan, these resistant improving substances are demonstrated to have incredible anti-tumor properties. While they don't straightforwardly cause the anti-tumor effect, they do trigger the bodies' own anti-tumor reaction. A type of anti-tumor white blood cell referred to as Natural Killer cells (NK cells) is produced by the body making the degree of NK cells in the body generally simple to quantify. At the point when human subjects are given Agari in their eating regimen, a 300% expansion of NK cells in the blood is seen inside 2-4 days. Natural killer cells are most popular for their ability to execute tumor cells before they become built up cancers, however there has additionally been proof for their job in controlling disease in the early periods of the safe reaction by the body.

Two Mushrooms Combine for Healthy Living

The Piedade mushroom, found in the rainforests of Brazil, is notable globally for its recuperating properties. Specifically, the people of the Piedade region who devoured this mushroom, were accounted for to have delighted in phenomenal health and life span, many living infections free a way into their 100s. Following a few clinical preliminaries, the Piedade mushroom and the Agaricusblazei mushroom, cultivated in the hilly region of California, were combined to shape a super-half breed and intense mushroom fluid. Utilizing a 10-phase extraction innovation that catches each nutritious component, and combined with Japanese Sasa Bamboo, an amazing antioxidant, this item is viewed as a powerhouse of supplements basic to keeping up and supporting a healthy and dynamic way of life. We never again need to go to the rainforest in Brazil or climb the mountains in California to find this unadulterated gold.

The Key Product Benefits

Each human is powerless to maturing, ecological contaminants, chemicals in nourishment and water, sickness and the worries of a quick paced way of life. Besides, we could all greatly profit by effectively improving our insusceptible systems. This combined mushroom item advances health and generally speaking prosperity. It builds natural killer cell activity, advances vitality and for the most part secures the body. It might likewise bring down cholesterol, control blood pressure and straightforwardness arteriosclerosis. Mushrooms are a wholesome dietary nourishment supplement with a functioning fixing demonstrated by research to be an effective improving operator to the invulnerable system.

Combined with your everyday admission of actuated fluid zeolite, a naturally framed mineral which strips the body of overwhelming metals and poisons, taking this mushroom item may solidly place you on the pathway to improved health by battling genuine health challenges. Just like the people of the Piedade region, you may proceed to live a healthy and upbeat life, getting a charge out of the enchantment of mushrooms.

For as far back as 20 years, Jannette has sought after her enthusiasm for health, prosperity and nature. She holds a Bachelor of Applied Science in Health Promotion and works with customers to improve their health and parts of personal advancement. She accepts that healthy eating, standard reflection, balance in all things and taking the right enhancements can make a tremendous improvement to the nature of our lives.

Mushrooms - Facts about This Magic Ingredient

Here are a couple of facts about Mushrooms, the enchantment fixing:

- ✓ Mushrooms are frequently named a vegetable or an herb, yet they are really fungi.
- ✓ While there are more than 14,000 mushrooms, just around 3,000 are eatable, around 700 have known medicinal properties, and less than one percent are perceived as noxious.
- ✓ People who gather mushrooms for utilization are known as mycophagists, and the demonstration of gathering them for such is known as mushroom chasing or simply "mushrooming".
- ✓ Only specimens that are freshly picked or appropriately saved ought to be consumed and not very old. When an eatable mushroom loses its freshness, bacterial provinces will form, and stomach upsets or more regrettable side effects can be normal if such specimens are ingested.
- ✓ The most ordinarily consumed mushroom in the world is Agaricusbisporus or the white catch mushroom. It has two different forms - Crimini or brown mushrooms with an increasingly earthy flavor and firmer texture, and Portabella mushrooms with a huge umbrella-molded top and meaty flavor.
- ✓ The Egyptians thought about mushrooms as a delicacy, and the Greeks accepted that mushrooms gave solidarity to warriors in fight. The Romans viewed mushrooms as a blessing from God and served them just

on merry events, while the Chinese loved them as a health nourishment.

- ✓ Mushrooms contain around 80 to 90 % water and are extremely low in calories (just 100 calories/oz). They have next to no sodium and fat and 8 to 10 % of the dry weight is fiber.
- ✓ Only about 45% of mushrooms produced are consumed in the fresh form. The remainder of the 55% is handled with 5% in the dehydrated form and 50% in the canned mushrooms form.
- ✓ This timeframe of realistic usability of mushrooms in the fresh form is short. Henceforth mushrooms are exchanged the world market for the most part in the prepared form.
- ✓ Some mushrooms produce exacerbates that battle cancer! This was found when researchers in Japan found that a network had bizarrely low cancer rates.
- ✓ Mushrooms can be used for coloring fleece and other natural strands. The chromophores of mushrooms are natural mixes and produce solid and distinctive hues, and all shades of the range can be accomplished with mushroom colors.

Causes of Anxiety Attacks - What You Must Know to Beat Anxiety

There are numerous causes of anxiety attacks, running from clinical issues to outside mental or passionate improvements. These causes are numerous and fluctuated and, in the event, that you are experiencing anxiety attacks, it is basic that you find out what is causing them.

1 - Hereditary Causes

Leading there might be your heredity fault. Anxiety attacks have been found to run in families, which leads numerous experts to reason that the characteristic can be found in the human genome. Then again, studies on hereditarily indistinguishable twins have shown that occasionally one twin will experience anxiety attacks, while the other won't. Another way where anxiety attacks can be acquired is through an excessively wary world view passed on by a patient's folks and the total pressure it causes.

2 - Biological Causes

There are likewise numerous biological causes to anxiety attacks, for example, inward ear unsettling influences (labyrinthitis), hyperthyroidism, hyperventilation disorder, hypoglycemia, prolapsed mitral valve (a heart infection), pheochromocytoma (an adrenal organ tumor), and Wilson's ailment (a hereditary issue). Indeed, even a nutrient B insufficiency caused by parasitic tapeworm disease or from a terrible eating routine can likewise cause anxiety attacks.

3 - Mental/Emotional Causes

Mental or intense subject matters can likewise trigger anxiety attacks. These incorporate summed up anxiety, fanatical urgent issue (OCD), fears, post horrible pressure issue (PTSD),significant personal misfortune, (for example, loss of a romantic accomplice), huge life changes, "imagine a scenario where" thinking, absence of self-assuredness, retained sentiments, mistaken convictions, and shirking of or relationship with anxiety-inciting circumstances or environs.

4 - Pharmalogical/Medicinal Causes

Pharmacological or medicinal causes incorporate amphetamines, liquor, marijuana, psilocybin (a hallucinogen found in certain mushrooms), symptoms from drugs, for example, Ritalin or different antidepressants (particularly toward the start or end of use), and energizers, for example, caffeine or nicotine. Some anxiety assault sufferers likewise build up an unreasonable dread of specific drugs, which may bring about anxiety attacks if they are taken, which is a simply psychosomatic effect like what placebos have been shown to produce.

As should be obvious, there are numerous causes of anxiety attacks, a large portion of which are totally out of your control in the event that you are having them. Fortunately, you can take care of business. The principal thing you have to comprehend is that it isn't your issue. Your anxiety attacks are nothing that you requested and not something that you fundamentally caused. If it is found that your anxiety attacks are caused by something outer that is effortlessly helped, your concern might be unraveled no problem at all. In the event that it is caused by a direction for living, for instance marijuana or liquor utilization, there are choices accessible. If it is something that is progressively ephemeral, at that point your emotional well-being proficient can guide you or potentially recommend drug that will assist you with dealing with your anxiety attacks.

Conclusion

Don't promptly accuse yourself or accept that there is simply a major issue with you if you are having anxiety attacks. If you look sufficiently hard, you will most likely have the option to find what the cause is. By and large, the cause of anxiety attacks can be immediately observed and managed by means of directing, medicine or self-improvement.

Far-Out Facts about Psychedelic Mushrooms

1. PSILOCYBIN ISN'T THE ONLY PSYCHEDELIC MUSHROOM

At the point when you state, "enchantment mushroom," a great many people think of Psilocybin. Psilocybin is a hallucinogenic compound found in excess of 75 species of mushrooms all through the world. Fresh or dried Psilocybin-containing mushrooms are eaten dried, fresh, or powdered into cases. It can likewise be synthesized in a lab.

While Psilocybin is certainly the most well-known compound in psychedelic mushrooms, it's not alone. Another psychedelic compound is muscimol. The Amanita Muscaria mushrooms (the notable red and white toadstool) are the most widely recognized wellspring of muscimol. You most likely know it as the mushroom emoticon on your iPhone.

With the two mushrooms, the portion, setting, and person are for the most part factors that influence results. They take twenty minutes to two hours to produce results and the trip will last 3 to 6 hours.

Mental effects incorporate uplifted tangible experiences and perceptual contortions (more brilliant hues, taste), mind flights, modified view of existence, an inability to recognize dream from reality, and the sky is the limit from there. Based on anecdotal evidence, Amanita Muscaria is said to frequently produce "darker" trips than "more joyful" Psilocybin.

2. PSYCHEDELIC MUSHROOMS HAVE BEEN UTILLLIZED FOR THOUSANDS OF YEARS

It's been a long, abnormal trip. Societies around the globe have used Psilocybin and Amanita Muscaria for both healing and spiritual growth for a long time.

There are 7,000-9,000-year old cavern works of art delineating mushrooms in Northern Algeria. In Central and South America, hallucinogenic mushrooms were viewed as god's substance, and along these lines exceptionally holy. In Siberia, Amanita Muscaria was utilized by Shamen in explicit ceremonies to speak with a greater soul and the dead.

While the long authentic use of anything doesn't mean it's good for humans, it's difficult to contend that "enchantment mushrooms" would not have an uncommon place with our progenitors.

3. PSILOCYBIN COULD BE A 'TRIP' TO JAIL

In the US, the possession, deal, and transport of Psilocybin are illegal. It is a Schedule 1 drug. Possession is an offense deserving of as long as a year in jail as well as $5,000 fee (short the legal advisor cost). Second offense turns into a lawful offense with a jail sentence of 3.5 years and $10,000 fee.

A fascinating caveat is that the possession of the mushrooms containing psilocybin isn't booked. Just the mixes themselves.

4. THERE'S ONE LEGAL PSYCHEDELIC MUSHROOM

While Psilocybin possession can have substantial legitimate issues, Amanita Muscaria doesn't. In fact, it is just illegal in Louisiana, the Netherlands, and Romania. It has rich social conventions in Siberia and Lapland, and based on persuading evidence, many trusts it assumes an important job in our present Christmas customs.

5. ARE PSYCHEDELIC MUSHROOMS SAFE?

There are no reasonable reports that Psilocybin-containing mushrooms are mentally or truly addictive. Their use does likewise not prompt reliance. Notwithstanding, with standard, repeated use of Psilocybin, resistance develops. Amanita Muscaria is additionally not addictive.

For Psilocybin, the middle deadly portion (LD) is about 17,000,000mg of dried mushroom with a 130lb person. Based on anecdotal evidence, the "ordinary portion" of dried Psilocybin mushroom people take is around 1,000-2,000mg. Along these lines, based on this information, it would appear to be practically difficult to ingest the LD.

For Amanita Muscaria, hypothetically, 15 tops could be a deadly portion. There are no dependably archived cases of death from Amanita Muscaria.

There is, notwithstanding, a high danger of misidentifying Amanita Muscaria, and it has fatal family members. Most mushroom-related deaths are as a result of two other Amanita mushrooms–relevantly named Death Cap and Destroying Angel mushrooms.

6. THERE ARE MANY POSSIBLE HEALTH BENEFITS

Psychedelic mushrooms appear to be leaving the woodwork and into the standard for a few reasons:

Spiritual Growth

Numerous psychedelic mushrooms lead to people having profound experiences feeling associated with the world and their god(s). In a twofold visually impaired examination at John Hopkins, over 50% of people rated the experience with Psilocybin to be the absolute most significant experience in their life (like the introduction of their first kid), and 1/3 rated it as top 5 spiritual experiences. While the genuine trip doesn't keep going long, clear recollections of this spiritual excursion appear to remain with you for any longer.

Creative Potential

Psilocybin is picking up footing in the start-up and business worlds to help calm thoughts of stress and self-analysis. People contend that it could assist you with keeping away from routine thought designs and can open your psyche to new thoughts. Lamentably, there isn't as of now much, assuming any, logical evidence to help this use-case.

Mood Stabilization

Researchers are starting to explore Psilocybin for treatment-safe despondency. For healthy people, it appears to expand constructive mood.

Alcohol and Smoking Cessation

While it might appear to be nonsensical, Psilocybin really shows guarantee in lessening dependence on alcohol and cigarettes.

Long-term Care

Psilocybin has likewise been given to mentally bothered cancer patients with despondency or anxiety. In two preliminaries at NYU and John Hopkins (one randomized twofold visually impaired, and the other randomized controlled), up to 80 percent report clinically noteworthy reductions in discouraged mood and anxiety following a half year.

Obviously, entangled or "awful" trips are not to be rejected. In these classes of health benefits and negative effects, considerably more research is required. In addition, notwithstanding the ongoing studies, Psilocybin is as yet illegal.

7. MICRODOSING IS A GOOD WAY TO START

While most research is done on genuinely high portions, microdosing is the way the vast majority start utilizing psychedelic mushrooms. Microdosing is taking a limited quantity of Psilocybin (100-300mg versus 1,000-2,000mg) normally, over a long timeframe and has as of late become famous. There isn't yet a lot of research on microdosing, so all evidence is absolutely anecdotal. There are currently in any event, microdosing retreats one can go on.

Microdosers report an increased mood, more vitality, no distrustfulness, or drowsy aftereffect frustration indications. It is not necessarily the case that in any event, microdosing is to be messed with. Research has been constrained because of the American War on Drugs, so we don't know all the results of long-term use... even on small scale sums.

At long last, recollect that clinical and healing uses of enchantment mushrooms are totally different than recreational uses of psychedelics. These are guided experiences, in an extremely controlled setting, with a specialist, shaman, or exceptionally proficient guide driving you through this excursion.

Fascinating Facts about Psilocybin Mushrooms

Is it reasonable to say that you are prepared to enter the captivating world of psilocybin mushrooms?

To start with, what are psilocybin mushrooms? They are a unique type of mushrooms (which are likewise called, all the more frequently, "magic mushrooms") which contain psychoactive mixes.

All the more explicitly, these little brown and white mushrooms can possibly totally change your point of view, both on the long-term and present moment, by encouraging a psychedelic experience.

This occurs because of their two primary psychoactive mixes, psilocybin and psilocin. People who were sufficiently gutsy to experience such an experience portray a wide scope of experiences, from mind flights to happiness, nausea or heaving.

Luckily, there are an ever-increasing number of clinical studies which demonstrate the fact that these mushrooms might be our partners towards a progressively healthy and healthy life.

Psilocybin Mushrooms Fact #1 – The "Magic Mushroom" Name Is Vague

Psilocybin mushrooms are not by any means the only psychoactive mushrooms out there. There is likewise Amanita Muscaria (the ruddy mushroom with white spots on it, which frequently shows up in fantasies) and Clavicepspurpurea (which is the fungus from which LSD was synthesized).

Every one of them are alluded to as "magic mushrooms" by a lion's share of psychonauts (adventurers of the human mind) in spite of the fact that their effects are totally unique.

Psilocybin Mushrooms Fact #2 – More Than 200 Species

You would think that there is only one type of psilocybin mushroom which is psychoactive and it's a simple as that – isn't that so? Indeed, for reasons unknown, there are around 200 species of mushrooms which can be named "magic mushrooms" (which means they have psychoactive mixes) – out of which a significant number of them are psilocybin mushrooms.

There is the classic Psilocybecubensis (Golden Teacher), Psilocybesemilanceata (Liberty Cap), Psilocybecyanescens (Wavy Cap), and some increasingly, each with their own "season" with regards to the real psychedelic experience.

Psilocybin Mushrooms Fact #3 – Psilocybin Mushrooms Is Legal in Several Countries

In spite of the fact that psilocybin mushrooms are illegal in many countries, there are some place it's legal to buy, expend, and even grow magic mushrooms.

In Holland, you can buy magic truffles (a previous phase of mushroom improvement) without overstepping the law. Numerous different countries, for example, Jamaica and Czech Republic, permit you to grow your own magic mushrooms.

Psilocybin Mushrooms Fact #4 – Psilocybin Mushrooms Are Considered Schedule 1 Drugs

The US is a lot harsher right now. Psilocybin mushrooms are viewed as Schedule 1 drugs (along with heroin and cocaine, which is an extremely inaccurate grouping to assemble these in a similar class).

This means the DEA considers psilocybin mushrooms to have a high potential for abuse and there are no acknowledged clinical uses, which makes it totally illegal to use.

Psilocybin Mushrooms Fact #5 – Psilocybin Mushrooms Are Not Addictive

Studies performed at Johns Hopkins University imply that psilocybin, one of the principle psychedelics fixing in psilocybin mushrooms, might be useful in defeating nicotine compulsion. Other comparable studies imply that they can likewise be used to treat anxiety, over the top habitual issue and other mental issue.

Psilocybin Mushrooms Fact #6 – They Dissolve the Control Mechanisms of The Brain

Practical MRIs performed during the psychedelic experience initiated by psilocybin mushrooms suggest that these "magic mushrooms" separate the typical control instruments of the brain, encouraging abnormal conditions of cognizance, and conceivably assisting with treating sorrow.

Psilocybin Mushrooms Fact #7 – Magic Mushrooms Have A Long History

Although Western development has as of late found the intensity of these psychoactive mushrooms, they have been around for a long period.

For thousands of years, psilocybin mushrooms have been used frequently in Central America for strict and spiritual functions. The Aztecs called psilocybin mushrooms "teonanacatl", which means "tissue of the divine beings".

The few stoneworks of art at Tassilin'Ajjer in Algeria created in the Mesolithic time frame are portraying the custom and stylized use of mushrooms.

Psilocybin Mushrooms Fact #8 – They Were Potentially Essential to Humanity's Evolution

There are numerous other entrancing hypotheses encompassing psilocybin mushrooms and some of them really bode well. For instance, a hypothesis set forward by American philosopher and psychonaut Terrence McKenna suggests that psilocybin mushrooms were basic in the mental and physical evolution of humanity.

He suggests that by eating Psilocybecubensis, a species of mushroom regularly found growing out of dairy animals' manure, Homo erectus grew better visual keenness and in this way turned out to be better trackers, which expanded our odds of endurance and evolution.

Psilocybin Mushrooms Fact #9 – They Induce Significant Spiritual Experiences

Another study done by Johns Hopkins University researched the spiritual effects of psilocybin. They were stunned by the outcomes.

Out of 36 guineas pigs, a third said that their experience was the hugest (spiritual) experience of their lives, while more than 66% expressed that it was certainly in their best five most noteworthy educational experiences.

All the more in this way, 79% of the subjects detailed expanded prosperity in the months following the study.

Psilocybin Mushrooms Fact #10 – You Can Grow Them at Home

You don't have to manage questionable people in obscure places to gain admittance to psilocybin mushrooms. Although still (actually) illegal in many countries, you can grow them in your own home easily, thus with greater genuine feelings of serenity and in full control of what you cultivate.

Starting to grow your psilocybin mushrooms can be as simple as requesting a growth unit on the web and simply watering it incidentally. Notwithstanding, it would be ideal if you ensure that you do practice alert in devouring these mind-changing mushrooms. These are not "toys" to mess with and they require accepting total accountability over your own experience.

Chapter 8

Psllocybe: The Species

There are some thirty thousand documented mushroom-producing fungi species around the world. Of these, it is known that around a hundred species or varieties contain psilocybin or related compounds. Most of these are found in the genera Psilocybe and Panaeolus, with some other genera appearing in Inocybe, Conocybe, Gymnopilusland. Not every species in these genera, of course, contains psilocybin, and even those who do may produce it in trace amounts only. We present methods for the cultivation of two types of psilocybin mushrooms in this book: the coprophilic (or dung-inhabiting) species Psilocybembensis, and the interrelated lignicolous (wood-inhabiting) species complex such as Psilocybeazurescens and P. cyanescens.

For several important reasons, we have chosen to focus on these particular species: they produce psilocybin in relatively high quantities, they have a long cultivation history and they fruit reliably under easily reproducible conditions. Additionally, they offer indoor (with P. cubensis) and outdoor (with any of the species in the P. azurescens complex) cultivation options. While there are certainly other well-known species which also meet these criteria, for any diligent grower the two types we have chosen should produce ample quantities of psilocybin. The goal of this chapter is to familiarize you with these animals, including their natural habitat, distribution, and behaviour, so you will understand their basic biology when you begin to work with them. This book is not meant to be a "field guide" and does not train you to identify and collect these wild species.

Foraging mushrooms, whether for food or psilocybin, requires a great deal of skill and knowledge. It is a true and potentially lethal danger to become contaminated as a result of misidentification. If you are interested in collecting your own mushrooms, we suggest you familiarize yourself with at least several good field guides (we've listed several excellent North American fungi guides in Appendix C) and consult with experts who already know your area's fungi directly. Chances are you have a local mycological club or society, where people can teach you what you need to know to identify wild mushrooms. Paul Stamets Psilocybin Mushrooms, if the Vl-orld is currently the most comprehensive text on the subject, is an essential addition to any mycology library for further reading about the many psilocybin-containing mushrooms found worldwide.

Psilocybecubensis

Psilocybecubensis is the most generally cultivated species of psychoactive mushrooms, for both recorded and biological reasons. Worldwide, it is one of the most widely recognized psilocybin containing species found in the wild, and subsequently among the most normally consumed and most notable. It is Psilocybecubensis fruiting from a plate of cased wheat berries. Additionally, one of the easiest to cultivate, since it fruits on a wide scope of substrates, and under an assortment of natural conditions. In spite of the fact that in the wild it grows solely on dung, under cultivation it will organic product from pretty much any substrate adequately high in carbon and nitrogen: oat straws, grains, grasses, com, even from wood, paper, or cardboard, whenever enhanced with some form of protein. Most mushroom species are very finicky in their growth and fruiting requirements, yet not P cubensis. This fact, combined with its sufficient potency, makes it probably the best specie for the beginner cultivator to grow.

We start with Psilocybe 3D shape/His because it is both the easiest to grow and the species of psilocybin-containing mushroom with which people are generally well-known. Its quickly developing, profoundly rhizomorphic mycelia, rich primordia, enormous, hearty fruits, and productive spore creation consolidate to make it among the most prototypical of Basidiomycetes. When you have worked with P cubensis for some time and have grown acquainted with the mushroom life cycle, you will be prepared to work with species that behave in increasingly unobtrusive ways. Psilocybecubensis is a skillet tropical mushroom that grows richly on the dung of cows, horses, and elephants, or on soils containing their manure. It tends to be found anyplace in the world with a wet, warm atmosphere, including Southeast Asia and Australia, India, Mexico, Central America, northern South America, and the Caribbean.

In the United States, it is normally found in the southeastern U.S. in the pre-summer and late spring, from Florida to the Texas Gulf Coast. It is among the biggest of psilocybin-containing species, with tops from I 12 to 5 crawls over, and thick stems up to 8 inches long. At the point when grown on grain or rice, it is typically unassumingly sized, however on manure or compost it can produce colossal, heavy fruits. It produces dull; purple-brown spore prints. At the point when taken care of, Psilocybecubensis frequently wounds profoundly blue. Albeit a bluing reaction regularly shows the presence of psilocybin in a mushroom, such evidence without anyone else can't be viewed as authoritative verification, since there are other disconnected parasitic exacerbates that behave correspondingly. In addition,' the nonattendance of the bluing reaction doesn't really preclude the presence of psilocybin-like atoms in a mushroom.

The bluing reaction occurs when psilocin oxidizes into an up 'til now uncharacterized dull blue chemical. Mushrooms containing low degrees of psilocin, yet noteworthy degrees of psilocybin, won't turn blue, in spite of their activity. P cubensis is considered moderately potent contrasted with other dynamic species. It can contain up to 1 .2% (dry weight) of psilocybin, psilocin, and baeocystin, with the normal some place around 0.5%, or 0.5mg/gram. While such averages are useful benchmarks for the correlation of the potency of one species to another, it is important to remember that potency can shift broadly among mushrooms of similar species. Certain strains, or a similar strain grown under contrasting conditions or on various substrates, can show exceptional variety in potency. Indeed, even a similar culture can shift starting with one flush then onto the next, with the second and third flushes ordinarily being the most potent.

The Woodloving Psilocybes

Despite the fact that Psilocybecubensis is anything but difficult to grow, there is one type of home cultivation to which it is ineffectively fit: the outside. In the wild, obviously, it grows outside, and it surely can be cultivated in a garden or wooded setting, however there is no genuine bit of leeway to doing as such. The two fundamental benefits of building up an outside mushroom garden is that it tends to be both lasting and furtive. You set it up in an off the beaten path place, forget about it until it fruits, reap the mushrooms, and afterward forget about it once more, until the procedure repeats itself the next year. When set up, a mystery mushroom fix ought to be pretty much self-continuing and totally unnoticeable with the exception of while fruiting. Psilocybecubensis doesn't possess all the necessary qualities for this kind of set-up, for a number of reasons. As a matter of first importance, it fruits quickly and consistently until its substrate is depleted of supplements and doesn't wait sufficiently long to be viewed as perpetual. Second, it grows on and fruits from a wide assortment of substrates, however, so do an entire host of other undesired life forms. Except if the fruiting substrate is kept clean (or possibly remarkably spotless), it will be colonized by molds and microscopic organisms long before the mushroom can turn out to be completely settled. That is the reason it is quite often grown inside under painstakingly controlled conditions. At last, being a tropical species, it doesn't grow well in cooler atmospheres and unquestionably can't endure the underneath frigid temperatures normal in numerous places throughout the winter months. Luckily for the future mushroom gardener, there are a number of different Psilocybes that are capable. These are the lignicolous, or wood-adoring, species, a gathering of related psilocybin-containing mushrooms that grow on wood chips or bark mulch and, attributable to their appearance, are on the whole known as the "caramel-topped" Psilocybes.

This gathering incorporates upwards of 10 species including Psilocybecyanescens, P azurescens, and P cyanofibrillosa, which are on the whole local to the Pacific Northwest of the United States, the Eastern European species P serbica and P bohemica, and P subaeruginosa and P tasmaniana, which are from Australia and New Zealand. In addition to their similitude in natural surroundings and appearance, these mushrooms all share another important trademark: they are among the most potent of the known psilocybin-containing species. Of these, Psilocybeazurescens, with its species designation implying the profound bluing reaction that occurs upon its dealing with, rules, containing P. cubensis. Different wood lovers are to some degree increasingly humble in potency, with detailed most extreme focuses in the 1 - 2% territory. All things considered, what the ligrucolous species of Psilocybes need wealth and stature when contrasted with Psilocybecubensis, they more than compensate for in quality, and a moderately little garden bed of only one of them can undoubtedly give enough psilocybin to keep going the gardener a long time, or if nothing else until the following year's fruiting. While these species are for the most part generally comparable in appearance, there are contrasts among them. In any case, under cultivation they all behave pretty much indistinguishably, and the techniques we give later in the book will work for any of them.

Psilocybecyanescens

Psilocybecyanescens is a moderately potent species usually found in the Pacific Northwest, from San Francisco to Canada. Its most unmistakable feature is an undulating top edge (the mycological term for the external edge of the top), which gives its mushrooms the epithet "wavy tops." It grows on wood chips or woody garbage in yards, garden beds, and along mulched pathways. At the point when young, its mushrooms have an unmistakable, cortinate ("web-like") halfway cover, which quickly disintegrates at development. P. cyanescens has a generally high psilocin substance, and blues immediately when wounded.

Psilocybeazurescens

Psilocybeazurescens is the most potent known Psilocybe mushroom. It is similar to P. cyanescens in appearance, then again, actually it comes up short on the last species' wavy edge, and frequently shows an articulated areola like knock on the focal point of its cap, a feature known as an umbo. In the wild, it grows ordinarily on wood garbage in sandy waterfront soils, frequently under ridge grasses. P. azurescens has an especially high baeocystin content, which may represent its purportedly special psychedelic "signature"; users regularly report that it produces a profound and unequivocally visionary effect, without noteworthy related physical inconvenience.

Psilocybecyanofibrillosa

Psilocybecyant fibrillosa is a small wood adoring Psilocybe normal to the Pacific shoreline of the U.S., from San Francisco to British Columbia. It isn't considered especially potent, containing just around 0.25% alkaloids by dried weight. In any case, there is evidence to suggest that a greater level of alkaloids is lost on drying this species than with others, making fresh P cyanif1brillosa specimens more potent than would be normal.

Psilocybebohemica

Psilocybebohemica is a central European relative of the North American lignicolousPsilocybes, found in Germany, Austria, and the Czech Republic. It is quite similar in appearance to P azurescens and P cyanofibrillosa and slightly less potent than P cyanescens, averaging around 1.1 % alkaloids by dried weight.

Psilocybesubaeruginosa

Psilocybesubaeruginosa is a relative of P Cyanescens and P Azurescens that is local to Tasmania and Australia. It is similar in appearance to P azurescens, however slightly smaller in stature, and its territory is tantamount to P cyanescens. Chemical studies of this species are restricted, however it is commonly viewed as a moderate to profoundly potent species, as it wounds profoundly blue on taking care of.

Copelandia / Panaeolus mushrooms

The Copelandia is a genus made out of 12 mushroom species, which are all known to contain the hallucinogens psilocin and psilocybin. American and European mycologists have consented to classify all members of the Copelandia genus under Panaeolus.

Mushrooms belonging to the Panaeolus genus are white to tan or gray, with long, slim delicate stems. They're dispersed in the tropics and neotropics of both hemispheres, growing in prairies, on dead moss, dead grass, sand ridges, rotted wood, and dung. Because of their psilocin content, they will in general wound and turn blue.

Delegate species under the Panaeolus genus are:

Panaeoluscambodginiensis. This is a potent hallucinogenic mushroom that contains psilocybin and psilocin. Its cap is under 23mm over, with a raised shape. The cap surface looks smooth with gray to dark gills. This is predictable with its spores which are likewise dark.

It grows on dung of water wild ox and was first found in Cambodia however end up being a broad species over the Asian subtropics and Hawaii.

Panaeoluscyanescens. This is another psilocybin mushroom belonging to the previously mentioned genus. Its cap is 1.5-4cm across with an incurved edge when young. Its shade is yellowish to brownish however it turns green or blue when harmed. Its spores are ebony.

It's likewise a dung-possessing species which frequents pastures in Africa, Australia, parts of Asia, North America, and South America.

Panaeolusbisporus. Genuinely, this species doesn't appear to be any unique from the P. cambodginiensis. It must be separated under a magnifying lens.

This little brown mushroom grows on dung and has dark spores. It's found in Hawaii, Southern California, North Africa, Spain, and Switzerland.

Panaeolustropicalis. This is among the most effective psilocybin mushrooms under the Copelandia/Panaeolus genus. The cap is clay-shaded, 1.5-2.5cm wide and is hemispheric to curved. The stem is 5-12cm long and turns blackish towards the base. It becomes blue when wounded.

Tropicalis additionally grows on dung and is regularly found in Hawaii, Central Africa, and Cambodia. It can likewise be seen growing in Mexico, Tanzania, the Philippines, Florida, and Japan

Inocybe mushrooms

Inocybe is a genus of mushroom-forming fungi. Members of Inocybe live in the underlying foundations of vascular host plants. Because of this, there are among the most exceptionally versatile types of mushrooms.

Run of the mill mushrooms under this genus are brown albeit a few species are lilac. Their caps are typically small and cone like, however straightening with age. Numerous caps have a particular smell, portrayed as spermatic or smelly.

Species under this genus are known to produce psychedelic effects.

Inocybeaeruginascens. The main example of this species was recorded on June 15, 1965. They're likewise widely distributed in temperate areas and has been accounted for in wet, sandy soils in central Europe and western North America.

These mushrooms are small with a conic to arched cap which is normally under 5cm in diameter. The cap shading changes from buff to light yellow brown, as a rule with greenish stains which vanish when the mushrooms dries. The spores are smooth and form a clay brown print.

They contain the psychoactive substances psilocybin, psilocin, baeocystin, just as a newfound substance which is named aeruginascin. Up until now, I. aeruginescens is the main type of magic mushrooms which produces aeruginascin.

Inocybecoelestium. This kind of magic mushroom is widely distributed in Europe. Its name "coelestium" means "celestials," the occupants of Mount Olympus. This is a gesture to its hallucinogenic properties.

Its physical attributes are commonly similar to most species under the Inocybe genus.

Inocybehaemacta. This species holds a solid similarity to the I. aeruginescens. This magic mushroom grows in beach front areas across Europe.

Inocybe tricolor. This individual from the Inocybe genus is distributed in temperate timberlands. It likewise contains both psilocybin and psilocin. It's found in Norway in central Europe. The cap is block red to chocolate brown, lighter towards the edge. It's typically 4cm across and produces spores which are ochre to tan brown.

Mycena mushrooms

This huge genus is made out of mushrooms which likewise grow on decaying matter. They are once in a while in excess of a couple of centimeters wide and are portrayed by a white spore print, a small bell-molded cap, and a thin delicate stem. Most mushrooms under the Mycena genus are brown or gray.

They are hard to recognize from other mushroom types and should be seen under a magnifying lens to separate. A few species are edible while other contain poisons. One of them contains the hallucinogen psilocybin.

Mycenacyanorrhiza. This is a small, white mushroom with a blue base. It's seen growing in forests on wood and leaves a white spore print.

It's reported to contain psilocybin, yet this is likely a bogus positive. Its edibility is debatable, and it doesn't have any verifiable record of being used as a hallucinogen.

Pluteus mushrooms. This genus contains more than 300 species that grow on wood or remains of wood. They leave pink spore prints and gills that are liberated from the stem.

A portion of these mushrooms are edible however the vast majority rate their taste and consistency as normal. A few members of this genus wound blue when taken care of, a sign that they contain psilocybin.

Pluteusbrunneidiscus. brunneidiscus is a species of agaric fungus initially found in Spain and the United States. It grows singularly on the wood of trees with wide leaves from June to November.

Pluteussalicinus. This European psychedelic mushroom grows on wood. It very well may be recognized by its silver-gray caps which range 2-8cm in diameter. It additionally has modest scopes close to the middle, darker at the edge, and is slightly translucent when clammy. The stem three to five centimeters long which is slightly swollen at the base.

The convergence of psilocybin and psilocin in dried examples of P. salicinus are reported within the scope of 0.21-0.35% and 0.011 and 0.05% individually.

Conocybe mushrooms

Most conocybe mushrooms types have long, thin, delicate stems and grow in ripe meadows on dead moss, dead grass, sand hills, rotted wood, and dung. Conocybe species are called cone heads because of their conical or bell-molded caps.

The conocybe genus contains at any rate 243 species of mushrooms, 4 of which contain the hallucinogenic mixes psilocin and psilocybin.

Conocybekehneriana. Not much is thought about this fungus but rather this species grows in Norway and Argentina. Its physical appearance is similar to the nonexclusive features of those belonging to the Conocybe genus.

Conocybesiligineoides. Otherwise called cone caps, this fungus is thin, small, and just around 3 crawls in stature. Its cap is bell-

formed with a rosy orange tint. At the point when spores form, it gets a corroded shading.

It's never observed in different parts of the world. All specimens were gathered in Mexico where it was initially reported as a hallowed mushroom used in healing and different ceremonies. They are ingested by local people either fresh or as tea.

Conocybecyanopus/Pholiotinacyanopus. This fungus is as of now assigned to the genus Pholiotina however was assigned to the Conocybe genus in 1935. It is a small mushroom that grows on decaying matter with a conic to extensively arched cap which is smooth and hued cinnamon brown.

It's generally small, typically under 25mm over, with striped edges. The stem is smooth and delicate with whitish areas at the base and brownish at the top. Its spores are additionally cinnamon brown. Most mycologists prompt against gathering and eating this species because of its solid likeness to harmful assortments.

Another attribute of this species is its capability to form sclerotia, a torpid form of the fruiting body which grows underground. Sclerotia are all the more commonly referred to as truffles.

This species grows in lawns, fields, and grassy parts in the temperate regions of North America, Austria, Belgium, Finland, France, Germany, Hungary, Denmark, Latvia, the Netherlands, Norway, Sweden, Switzerland, Poland, Russia, Ukraine, and the United States.

Conocybesmithii/Pholiotinasmithii. Similar to the species referenced over, it's presently renamed into the Pholiotina genus.

The P. smithii is found in North America and regularly grows in lowlands, trench and swampy areas, commonly in sphagnum moss. It's additionally found along waterway banks and in lawns. It is known to occur in Canada, Oregon, Wisconsin, Washington, and on antiquated man-made earthen hills in Northern Michigan. It fruits in late spring. Smithii's caps are 0.3-1cm across with a conic to raised shape which grows to about level with age. Its cinnamon-brown shading is reliable with the tone of its spores.

Regardless of its gentle hallucinogenic effects, specialists firmly exhort against utilizing them for psychedelic analyses because of their similarities with noxious mushrooms.

Psilocybemexicana alludes to a species of mushroom that grows locally in Central and South America. These mushrooms have been used for thousands of years by indigenous people.

Psilocybemexicana

Psilocybemexicana is fundamentally the same as in appearance to semilanceata. They have huge caps (normally extending from 10-20mm) with a conical or bell shape. They may have a slight papilla (or umbo) and are generally light brown or beige in shading. Like semilanceata, these mushrooms may feature blue or greenish tones, and effectively turn blue when harmed.

Psilocybemexicana can grow single or in gatherings. It likes to spring up among moss on side of the road and trails, moist glades, or the grassy areas of forests. These mushrooms are normally found at heights between 300–550 meters among May and October.

Psilocybesemilanceata,

Psilocybesemilanceata, otherwise called "freedom caps," are believed to be one of the most potent kinds of psilocybin mushroom. They are portrayed by their large, leathery-brown caps and pale, bended stems.

The caps of these mushrooms possess a diameter between 5-22mm and a length of approximately 6-22mm. They can be either conical or bell-molded; the cap can differ in shading depending on the hydration of the mushroom. All around hydrated caps will show darker shades of brown (sometimes with a blue or greenish tinge) and may have grooves running down them, relating to the gills on the underside. On the underside of the cap, Psilocybesemilanceata will have between 15-27 restricted gills. At the point when harmed, these mushrooms rapidly turn blue.

Psilocybesemilanceata can be found across both North America and Europe. It tends to grow in knolls and fields, particularly. However, they don't grow legitimately out of dung like some different species.

PsilocybeAzurescens

Otherwise called the "flying saucer mushroom," PsilocybeAzurescens is a very potent species of magic mushroom. It is believed to grow naturally, just along a small area of the West Coast of the United States. In spite of the fact that, it has since been cultivated in numerous countries around the world.

As the name suggests, azurescens tend to have large, saucer-like caps going from 30-100mm in diameter. Younger mushrooms may have slightly progressively conic caps that in the long run level with development. At the point when damp, these mushrooms are commonly chestnut or caramel brown in shading and when developed, may show dim blue (practically dark ish) tints. The edges of the caps may have slight scores that compare with the gill's underneath. Wounded areas of the mushroom tend to turn dull blue rapidly. Develop azurescens will have dim gills and chalk-white stems.

These mushrooms ordinarily grow in bunches in wood chips as well as sandy soils. They particularly like waterfront areas and tend to spring up around ridge grasses among September and January.

Psilocybebaeocystis

Psilocybebaeocystis are known by an assortment of names, including "bottle caps," "bumpy tops," "blue bells," and "olive caps." They are generally found in the US over the Pacific Northwest. These mushrooms regularly have medium-sized caps estimating between 15-55mm. The caps have a conical shape and are normally thin and unmistakably undulated because of the gill's underneath.

They have a remarkable shading, displaying a dull, olive brown tone, sometimes with steel blue tinges. The stems are long, can be straight or bended, and are generally chalk-white in appearance.

Baeocystis mushrooms wound effectively, so, all things considered they normally recolor blue. They love growing in conifer mulch, wood chips, or potentially lawns wealthy in lignin. They sometimes additionally grow from the fallen cones of Douglas fir. They tend to be found growing under different plants like rhododendrons and flower hedges in mulched garden beds.

This is what Magic Mushrooms Do to Your Body and Brain

Evidence tripping on magic mushrooms could in reality free the mind. A few studies, including two promising ongoing clinical preliminaries, suggest that psilocybin - shrooms' psychoactive fixing - may hold the potential to help soothe serious anxiety and depression.

Here are a couple of the ways we know shrooms can influence your brain and body:

Shrooms can cause you to feel good.

As indicated by the National Institute on Drug Abuse, magic mushrooms can prompt feelings of unwinding that are similar to the effects of low dosages of marijuana.

Like other hallucinogenic drugs, for example, LSD or peyote, shrooms are thought to produce the majority of their effects by following up on neural highways in the brain that use the synapse serotonin, as per the National Institute on Drug Abuse.

All the more explicitly, magic mushrooms influence the brain's prefrontal cortex, some portion of the brain that directs theoretical thinking, thought investigation, and assumes a key job in mood and observation.

A five-year study of the drug suggests it could work "like a careful intercession" for dysfunctional behavior.

Results from two controlled clinical preliminaries of the effects of psilocybin on patients dealing with depression and trouble identified with confronting the finish of life suggest that a solitary portion of the drug would one be able today be an integral asset for treating depression and anxiety.

The first was done by researchers from Johns Hopkins University, the other by researchers at New York University.

A half year after the experience, 80 percent of the Johns Hopkins members indicated noteworthy abatements in side effects of depression and anxiety, as estimated by what's viewed as a highest quality level mental assessment.

The NYU team says that between 60 percent and 80 percent of its members had similarly decreased anxiety and depression 6.5 months after a solitary psychedelic trip.

A few researchers think shrooms could likewise help soothe anxiety after they're used.

In any case, you may likewise feel on edge - at any rate while you're on the drug.

In a significant number of the case reports from the NYU study, participants reported encountering extraordinary anxiety and distress - running from a couple of moments to a couple of hours - during their trip.

It was just a while later that some said they started to feel a sense of alleviation; and even this experience may fluctuate essentially for every person.

Your pupils may likewise dilate.

Expanded degrees of serotonin, which can be an aftereffect of utilizing shrooms, can dilate your pupils.

What's more, your sense of time may be twisted.

Feeling just as time has been eased back down is one of the symptoms of utilizing shrooms, as per the National Institute on Drug Abuse.

You may have an out-of-body experience.

Shrooms can prompt experiences that appear to be genuine yet aren't.

These types of out-of-body experiences, in which users may watch a rendition of themselves, ordinarily start 20 to an hour and a half in the wake of ingesting the drug and can keep going up to 12 hours, as indicated by the National Institute on Drug Abuse.

Experiences can shift based on the amount you take, just as by your personality, your mood and even your environment.

Furthermore, you may feel increasingly open or imaginative.

After Johns Hopkins clinicians initiated out of body experiences in a small gathering of healthy volunteers dosed with psilocybin, the members said they felt progressively open, increasingly imaginative, and increasingly keen to excellence.

At the point when the researchers caught up with the volunteers a year later, almost 66% said the experience had been one of the most important in their lives; near half kept on scoring higher on a personality trial of openness than they had before taking the drug.

A few users have reported waiting illusory observations that might be linked with an uncommon issue called HPPD.

Since the 1960s, there have been dispersed reports of something called hallucinogen enduring observation issue - when mental trips proceed with long after somebody's taken a hallucinogenic drug, commonly LSD.

(There are additionally some anecdotal reports of it from people who've used shrooms).

Researchers despite everything still can't seem to think of a severe meaning of HPPD, yet John Halpern, an associate educator of psychiatry at Harvard Medical School and lead creator of the latest audit of HPPD, told the New Yorker that:

"It appears to be inescapable", based on 20 related studies going back to 1966, "that probably a few people who have used LSD, specifically, experience relentless perceptual variations from the norm suggestive of intense inebriation, worse inferable from another clinical or mental condition."

Chapter 9

What is the nutritional value of mushrooms?

Mushrooms are edible fungus that can give a few important supplements. The numerous kinds of mushroom have differing creations and nourishing profiles.

Right now, about the dietary substance and conceivable health benefits of eating mushrooms. We additionally give a few hints on planning and serving them and depict the risks.

Health benefits

Mushrooms contain protein, vitamins, minerals, and antioxidants. These can have different health benefits.

For instance, antioxidants are chemicals that help the body wipe out free radicals. Free radicals are dangerous results of digestion and other real procedures. They can amass in the body, and if too some gather, oxidative pressure can result. This can hurt the body's cells and may prompt different health conditions.

Among the antioxidant operators in mushrooms are:

- selenium
- vitamin C
- choline

Cancer

The antioxidant content in mushrooms may help prevent lung, prostate, breast, and different types of cancer, as indicated by the National Cancer Institute.

A few sources have suggested that selenium may help prevent cancer, yet a Cochrane audit, from 2017, found no evidence to affirm this.

Mushrooms additionally contain a small measure of vitamin D. There is some evidence that vitamin D supplementation may help prevent or treat a few kinds of cancer, however as indicated by a 2018 report, the effect may differ from person to person.

Choline is another antioxidant in mushrooms. A few studies have suggested that consuming choline can reduce the risk of certain types of cancer, however at any rate one other study has demonstrated that it might expand the risk of prostate cancer.

It is significant that consuming a supplement as an enhancement isn't equivalent to consuming it in the diet.

What links are there among cancer and the diet?

Diabetes

Dietary fiber may help deal with a number of health conditions, including type 2 diabetes.

A 2018 audit of meta-examinations reasoned that people who eat a ton of fiber may have a lower risk of creating type 2 diabetes. For the individuals who as of now have it, fiber may help reduce blood glucose levels.

A cup of cut, crude mushrooms, gauging 70 grams (g), gives very nearly 1 g of fiber.

The Dietary Guidelines for Americans suggest that grown-ups expend 22.4–33.6 g of dietary fiber every day, depending on sex and age.

Mushrooms, beans, a few vegetables, brown rice, and entire grain foods would all be able to contribute to a person's day by day prerequisite of fiber.

Attempt our 7-day diabetes meal plan.

Heart health

The fiber, potassium, and vitamin C in mushrooms may contribute to cardiovascular health.

Potassium can help direct blood pressure, and this may diminish the risk of hypertension and cardiovascular malady. The American Heart Association (AHA) prescribe lessening the admission of included salt in the diet and eating more foods that contain potassium.

As indicated by current rules, people ought to expend around 4,700 milligrams (mg) of potassium every day. Mushrooms show up on the AHA's rundown of foods that give potassium.

A 2016 study reasoned that people with a vitamin C inadequacy were bound to experience cardiovascular infection and suggested that consuming vitamin C may help prevent this disease. They didn't find evidence that vitamin C enhancements can reduce the risk of this type of ailment.

There is some evidence that consuming a type of fiber called beta-glucans may bring down blood cholesterol levels. Beta-glucans occur in the cell dividers of numerous kinds of mushrooms.

The stem of the shiitake mushrooms is a good wellspring of beta-glucans.

The Mediterranean diet incorporates a scope of plant foods, for example, mushrooms.

In pregnancy

Numerous women take folic corrosive, or folate, supplements during pregnancy to help fetal health, however mushrooms can likewise give folate.

A cup of entire, raw mushrooms contains 16.3 micrograms (mcg) of folate. Current rules prescribe that grown-ups expend 400 mcg of folate every day.

What foods would it be advisable for you to eat and abstain from during pregnancy?

Different benefits

Mushrooms are plentiful in B vitamins, for example,

- riboflavin, or B-2
- folate, or B-9
- thiamine, or B-1
- pantothenic corrosive, or B-5
- niacin, or B-3

B vitamins help the body get vitality from nourishment and form red blood cells. A number of B vitamins likewise seem, by all accounts, to be important for a healthy brain.

The choline in mushrooms can help with muscle development, learning, and memory. Choline helps with keeping up the structure of cell layers and assumes a job in the transmission of nerve driving forces.

Mushrooms are likewise the main veggie lover, nonfortified dietary wellspring of vitamin D.

A few different minerals that might be hard to get from a vegetarian diet —, for example, selenium, potassium, copper, iron, and phosphorus — are accessible in mushrooms.

Healthful substance

Numerous types of mushroom are edible, and most give about similar quantities of similar supplements per serving, paying little mind to their shape or size.

The table underneath shows the amount of every supplement a 96-g cup of entire, raw mushrooms gives. It likewise shows the amount of every supplement grown-ups ought to devour each day, depending on their sex and age.

Mushrooms additionally contain a number of B vitamins, including thiamine, riboflavin, B-6, and B-12.

Tips for getting ready mushrooms

There are around 2,000 edible assortments of mushrooms, yet just a bunch are accessible on the American market.

They include:

- white, or "button"
- brown cremini
- portobello
- shiitake
- oyster
- wood ear
- enoki

Regular assortments accessible at rancher's business sectors and some markets include:

- morel
- chanterelle

A few people pick wild mushrooms, however it is fundamental to realize which are edible, as some contain fatal poisons.

Tips for buying

- ✓ When buying fresh mushrooms, picked ones that are firm, dry, and unbruised. Maintain a strategic distance from mushrooms that seem foul or wilted.
- ✓ Store mushrooms in the fridge. A person ought not wash or trim them until the time has come to cook with them.
- ✓ A wide scope of mushroom items is accessible for buy on the web.

Tips for serving

- ✓ The Environmental Working Group, which surveys foods for their pesticide substance, placed mushrooms that grow in the U.S. in its 2019 rundown of the 15 cleanest foods, alluding to generally low hints of pesticides.
- ✓ However, people should in any case wash and clean them cautiously before utilizing them to expel any soil and coarseness. If important, trim the parts of the bargains. You can use mushrooms entire, cut, or diced.

To incorporate more mushrooms into the diet, attempt:

- sautéing any type of mushroom with onions for a fast, delicious side dish
- adding mushrooms to pan-sears
- topping a serving of mixed greens with raw, cut cremini or white mushrooms
- stuffing and heating portobello mushrooms
- adding cut mushrooms to omelets, breakfast scrambles, pizzas, and quiches

- sautéing shiitake mushrooms in olive oil or juices for a healthful side dish
- removing the stems of portobello mushrooms, marinating the caps in a blend of olive oil, onion, garlic, and vinegar for 60 minutes, at that point barbecuing them for 10 minutes
- adding flame broiled portobello mushrooms to sandwiches or wraps

To get ready dried mushrooms, leave them in water for a few hours until they are delicate.

Possible health risks

Wild mushrooms can make a scrumptious dish, yet the poisons in certain mushrooms can trigger deadly health issues. Some wild mushrooms additionally contain significant levels of overwhelming metals and other destructive chemicals.

To maintain a strategic distance from these threats, just devour mushrooms from a reliable source.

Takeaway

Mushrooms can be a healthful addition to a shifted diet. They are anything but difficult to plan and give a scope of supplements.

People should just eat mushrooms from a reliable source, as certain types are poisonous.

Street names for psilocybin

Drug vendors seldom sell psilocybin under its real name. Instead, the drug might be sold as:

- magic mushrooms
- shrooms
- boomers
- zoomers

- mushies
- simple Simon
- little smoke
- sacred mushrooms
- purple energy
- mushroom soup
- cubes

Effects Share on Pinter

The effects of psilocybin are commonly similar to those of LSD.

They incorporate an adjusted view of time and space and exceptional changes in mood and feeling.

Potential effects of psilocybin include:

- euphoria
- peacefulness
- spiritual arousing
- quickly changing feelings
- derealization, or the feeling that your surroundings are not real
- depersonalization, or a fantasy like sense of being separated from your surroundings
- distorted thinking
- visual modification and twisting, for example, radiances of light and distinctive hues
- dilated pupils
- dizziness
- drowsiness
- impaired focus
- muscle shortcoming

- lack of coordination
- unusual body sensations
- nausea
- paranoia
- confusion
- frightening pipedreams
- vomiting
- yawning

The effects of psilocybin shift between people, based on contrasts in the psychological state and personality of the user and the prompt condition.

In the event that the recreational user experiences issues with psychological wellness or feels on edge about utilizing the hallucinogen, they face a higher risk of having a terrible experience.

Mental misery is the unfriendly occasion frequently reported after recreational use of psilocybin. This misery can appear as outrageous anxiety or transient psychosis.

Chapter 10

Psilocybin as a treatment for depression

Conversations are on-going if psychological specialists can use psilocybin and similar hallucinogens as a treatment for depression.

Two extremely ongoing studies have taken a gander at psilocybin as a treatment. One study inspected the ability of psilocybin to reduce depression symptoms without dulling feelings, and the other surveyed the connection between any positive helpful results and the idea of psilocybin-prompted hallucinations.

While a few researchers are investigating some helpful uses for psilocybin, they still, at present, view psilocybin as perilous and illegal.

Risks

People who have taken psilocybin in uncontrolled settings may take part in crazy behavior, for example, driving while inebriated.

A few people may experience tireless, upsetting modifications to the way they see the world. These effects are frequently visual and can last from anyplace from weeks to years subsequent to utilizing the hallucinogen.

Doctors presently analyze this condition as hallucinogen continuing perception disorder (HPPD), otherwise called a flashback. A flashback is an awful review of a seriously upsetting experience. The memory of this upsetting experience during hallucinogen use would be an awful trip, or a mind flight that takes an upsetting turn.

A few individuals experience more disagreeable effects than hallucinations, for example, dread, fomentation, confusion, delirium, psychosis, and disorders that take after schizophrenia, requiring a trip to the emergency room.

As a rule, a specialist will treat these effects with medicine, for example, benzodiazepines. These effects regularly resolve in 6 to 8 hours as the effects of the drug wear off.

At long last, however the risk is small, some psilocybin users risk incidental poisoning from eating a poisonous mushroom by mistake.

Symptoms of mushroom poisoning may incorporate muscle spasms, confusion, and delirium. Visit an emergency room promptly if these symptoms occur.

Because hallucinogenic and different poisonous mushrooms are basic to most living conditions, a person ought to consistently expel all mushrooms from areas where kids are routinely present to prevent inadvertent utilization.

Most coincidental mushroom ingestion results in minor gastrointestinal disease, with just the most extreme cases requiring clinical consideration.

Abuse potential

Psilocybin isn't chemically addictive, and no physical symptoms occur in the wake of halting use.

However, standard use can cause a person to get tolerant to the effects of psilocybin. Cross-resilience likewise occurs with different drugs, including LSD and mescaline. People who use these drugs must hold up at any rate a few days between dosages to experience the full effect.

Following a few days of psilocybin use, individuals may potentially experience mental withdrawal and experience issues changing in accordance with reality.

Fungi: Mushroom

Mushrooms are among the strangest plants on earth. The word mushroom is thought to get from an Old French word, mousseron, signifying "moss grower." They spring up obviously all of a sudden medium-term and vanish almost as fast. Their growth propensities were not surely known as of not long ago. Some glimmer around evening time with a green brightness. Numerous fungi grow in ever-extending circles. Some dangerous mushrooms have long been a piece of certain mystery customs, giving mind-adjusting substances. Subsequently mushrooms have been adored as doorways to different measurements that solitary the users are favored to visit. One scholar, John Allegro, in The Sacred Mushroom and the Cross, states that the Egyptian mushroom pictograph, long believed to speak to a kind of parasol, really speaks to the harmful Amanita Muscaria mushroom, which in its beginning periods of poisoning causes splendid hallucinations. The mushroom is phallic in appearance and is "conceived" from a volva that resembles an egg. Allegro thinks that there has existed all through the ages a mushroom cult—and that the Christ figure really advanced from this crude fertility cult. The word toadstool, however, colorfully suggestive, alludes for the most part to any mushroom that is poisonous. To rummage for mushrooms, you will require good mushroom field guides.

Choose one with drawings or tinted lithographs, and another with good photos of the mushrooms, for there are poisonous mushrooms that can execute you. In any case, my way of thinking about that is similar to my philosophy about poisonous snakes and Lyme-ailment conveying ticks: You don't stay out of the woods because there are things in there that may hurt you; you simply continue with alert and mindfulness. On account of fungi, stay with the sheltered ones. Fungi like wet weather, wet wood, and wet woods. They need chlorophyll, which is the green-making chemical found in plants, and they prosper in heat and sogginess. There are thousands of various types of mushrooms, and thousands additional fungi, a tremendous gathering without which we were unable to live, including everything from the yeast that raises our bread to the brute that gives you competitor's foot. If you need to test mushrooms that are not depicted in this for wellbeing, above and beyond is to make a spore print, a basic procedure that I regularly use to recognize new fungi. All you need is a pack of dark development paper and ordinary white paper. To make a spore print, lay a bit of dark paper slightly covering a white one. At that point lay an open mushroom, gills down, over the line where the dark paper and white paper meet, with the goal that its spores will fall half on white paper and half on dark. Spread the mushroom with an upside-down bowl and leave it for two to eight hours. At that point look at the spores. Contrast them and what your books state; all mushroom books recognize the color of the spore print. The spores will store on the two colors of paper, and the difference will permit you to see the nuance of the spore color. A level bottomed bin for social affair keeps mushrooms fit as a fiddle, however a basic food item pack or plastic sack will do. You can practically tell from your specimens which ones need extraordinary spoiling and which are good to hurl into a plastic sack.

Mushrooms sometimes get negative criticism because of the unsafe assortments. However, good mushrooms, if you stay with those easy to distinguish, are almost without calorie, pose a flavor like the woodland air smells after rain, are easy to find, and make scrumptious meatless gourmet dishes. In all the mushroom plans, any mushroom can really be fill in for some other. Also, by and by, measures of the mushroom are not urgent. Mushrooms (and eggplant) are the most noticeably terrible offenders for absorbing oil and margarine. Have a go at brushing them lightly with oil or softened margarine and broiling them in the broiler for a similar effect.

Morels

Morels (Morchellaappalachiensis, M. esculenta, M. angusticeps, M. deliciosa, M. crassipes) are perhaps the most delightful wild mushrooms, and once distinguished, difficult to confuse with any others. Morchella is simply the Latin term for "mushroom," and esculenta and deliciosa imply that one is "edible" and the other "delightful." Angusticeps means "tight," and Appalachians is the name of the subspecies that grows in the Appalachian Mountains from Newfoundland to Georgia; mycologists vary on whether it is an alternate subspecies from angusticeps. Morels, mainstream all through the Temperate Zone here and in Europe, pass by different folk names. They are called land fish or upland fish (maybe from their shape, maybe from their subtle flavor, which I would call earthy yet which some may call fishy); marls (without a doubt a corruption of the name, yet in addition possibly after the kind of delicate, brittle stone geologists call marl, which is loaded with openings and pits like the fungi); merkles, which some think is a corruption of "supernatural occurrences"; smokies (the dark ones); honeycomb mushrooms; wipe mushrooms; mushrooms, which one accept originates from a folksy mishearing; and morchellas, from the Latin name. There is a dark morel, running in color from gray to tan to corroded brown, a pale brilliant one, and a grayish white one. All are fine to eat

Description, Habitat, and Season

Despite the fact that the dark ones (M. angusticeps and M. appalachiensis) seem half a month sooner than the lighter ones, they cover, and most "messes" will have specimens of a few kinds, including one that might possibly be a genuine morel, yet resembles the others, M. semilibra, or the sans half morel (supposed because the cap appends to the stalk halfway down the cap). It is additionally edible. Morels spring up in hardwood forests highly involved with spring "when the oak leaves are the size of mouse ears," and are said to be particularly various in years and places following a timberland fire. Where you find jack-in-the-platforms and trillium, search for morels. Some assortment grows wherever north of the Tropics right to the Arctic Circle.

All morels have the trademark appearance differently depicted as hollowed, furrowed, spongelike, cone-molded, or wrinkled; all are somewhere in the range of three and six inches high; all have empty stems and empty insides; and all are formed enigmatically like trees. They have no gills. None of them is easy to see on the woodland floor. The flavor is totally flawless: smoky, earthy, tricky, etch mushroom! A flat basket is most likely the best thing to take picking, for it keeps the sensitive morels unblemished superior to anything basic food item sacks or plastic packs. However, a flat basket is clumsy, and I select rather for the comfort of a red plastic tote. (Red can be seen from a separation, and you can use it to check a chasing limit while you are hovering searching for mushrooms.)

{ Recipes }

As morels are empty, they need uncommon cleaning treatment. Cut each in half from top to bottom to determine in the event that it houses any insalubrious creatures: I've found stones, centipedes, and slugs inside morels, so be cautioned. At that point bump them in warm, vigorously salted water for around 5 minutes (this removes any soil sections that might be trapped in the wrinkled surface) before draining the parts on paper towels. The salt will drive out the minor wood insects that likewise call these mushrooms home. There are a few ways to keep morels. Obviously, they are best used fresh, as most things seem to be. However, when cooked, they can be solidified. A few folks' dry morels by sewing them onto a string and placing them in a warm, dry stove or storage room until they are thoroughly dry or utilizing a dehydrator.

Puffballs

Puffball, like such a significant number of folk names for wild foods, portrays this fungus well: a puffy ball. This fungus belongs to a few related species. Its most normal genus name, Calvatia, originates from the Latin word calva, signifying "scalp," "uncovered head," or even "skull," which apropos portrays this round, whitish fungus. The western puffball, Calbovistasubsculpta, has bovis in the name, maybe suggesting its propensity to grow in dairy animals' fields; subsculpta depicts the curious cut effect of the surface.

Description, Habitat, and Season

Puffballs grow everywhere throughout the world in temperate zones, in the spring or in wet summer weather, however frequently they spring up medium-term in the late summer, after rain, in fields. They like fairways, lawns, and fields, and they come back to similar areas consistently. Puffballs shift gigantically in size, at their smallest like round white golf balls, and at their largest like round lightly browned portions of bread, six to eight creeps across. They are pure white all through, with no gill structure, and are firm and foamlike inside, something like thick fluffy cake in both weight and consistency. One western species has flattish, cone like scales covering the surface. Toss out any that are not pure white all through, that smell like wet pooch, or that have weaknesses, worm gaps, or insects in them. Puffballs can be securely gathered in baskets or packs. When home, they need a brisk wash to get any earth off the external surfaces. Always cut small puffballs through from top to bottom to make sure they are white all through. Since Amanita, lethal poisonous white-gilled mushrooms, do frequently grow among different mushrooms, be certain you haven't unintentionally gotten the catch form of an Amanita. In the event that you have, you will plainly observe the diagram of the gill structure, stalk, shroud, and cap. Obviously you should dispose of that example and wash your blade a long time before going on to the following mushroom.

{ Recipes }

If the mushrooms are a firm, strong white "wipe" all through, at that point they can be sliced, diced, or slashed, and sautéed gradually, or sliced and brushed with oil or liquefied margarine and heated until brown. They can be solidified subsequent to cooking for some time in the future if there are beyond any reasonable amount to eat immediately. I have never known about anybody attempting to dry puffballs, however in principle it should be conceivable, in the event that you cut them thin.

Chanterelles

Chanterelles (Cantharelluscibarius) are midsummer wet-weather mushrooms that can be seen from far off. The Latin name of the genus, Cantharellus, originates from cantharus, "a drinking cup," and along these lines characterizes the shape splendidly. The dark chanterelle is undoubtedly suggestive fit as a fiddle of a cornucopia, whose name gets from the word for horn in Latin. Different kinds are awesome.

Description, Habitat, and Season

Chanterelles have fluted edges, are shaped like flared wineglasses or containers, and in place of gills underneath have veins. Chanterelles come in numerous colors. The easiest to see, C. cibarius, are egg-yolk yellow and appear as though flowers sprouting on the backwoods floor. There are additionally white chanterelles in New England woods called C. subalbidus, or "practically white," and dark or gray chanterelles called Craterelluscornucopioides, which describes the fungi as both "crated" and "cornucopia-shaped." These are called likewise death trumpets; however, they are tasty and safe. There is a gray-purple-brown chanterelle called Cantharellusclavatuswhich means "club-shaped," from the Latin clavus), and small red orange, or cinnabar, chanterelles called Cantharelluscinnabarinus. These mushrooms, like most others, spread by underground mycelia (little white strings you sometimes observe hanging off the bottoms), so look without fail in a similar territory where you found them once. I have found chanterelles regularly in coniferous, particularly pine, woods, a day to three days after a good absorbing rain midsummer. Of course, a basket with a wide bottom would be ideal, yet a flat-bottomed sack, or even a plastic pack, will do

{ Recipes }

Gather just the young mushrooms. Insects additionally find chanterelles flavorful, and since you don't have any desire to destroy your bunch with one bug-invaded example, check for bug pervasion by cutting the stem off halfway between the veins and the soil and checking the stem. In the event that it has bug burrows, dispose of the example.

BEEFSTEAK MUSHROOM

This is one of my preferred pre-fall mushrooms. Beefsteak mushroom (Fistulina hepatica) looks on the top rather like raw liver (which its Latin name reflects) or a bit of steak, and it grows shelf like out from old logs or stumps, particularly oak and chestnut.

Description, Habitat, and Season

Beefsteak mushroom sometimes even "drains" when cut. It looks whitish or pinkish underneath, however if you take a gander at it with an amplifying glass, you will see that the underside is made up of swarmed fistulas, or small separate cylinders. Most pieces will be about the size of a hand. Beefsteak mushroom has a sourish meaty taste and a pleasant chewy consistency, and it grows all through the mid-year if it's wet. Hold out one hand, at that point run your other hand over the top, seeing how the skin appears to be free. Beefsteak mushroom has a similar feel, caused by a gelatinous layer simply under the surface. Use it the way you'd use some other mushroom.

Sulfur Shelf

The name Polyporussulphureus tells anybody with even a smattering of Latin this is a many-pored mushroom of a yellow tone. The normal name, sulfur rack mushroom, describes its growth design, out from the trunk of a tree like a heap of racks, just as its sulfur yellow color. This is sometimes called the chicken mushroom: The tissue is genuinely dry and thick, and it tastes a lot of like chicken breast.

Description, Habitat, and Season

Polyporussulphureus are easy to recognize: They grow in midsummer on the sides of hardwood trees or on spoiling logs are sunset orange-colored on top, with fluted edges and yellow, permeable bottoms instead of gills. Sulfur rack fungi sometimes grow to tremendous size, with sections climbing numerous feet up on a tree. However, if the ones you find are big, take just the smallest, freshest sections, or the external edges, for the more seasoned part nearer to the tree can be intense and solid enhanced, also loaded with bugs. These fungi aren't as delicate as most, so they needn't be treated with as a lot of delicacy. Simply take them home, cautiously forget about and flush all earth, and drain until dry on paper towels.

{ Recipes }

Sulfur rack mushrooms are ideal, I think, creamed. They need thin cutting and moderate cooking or sautéing, as they are harder than most mushrooms. However, they have a magnificent flavor.

Oyster Mushrooms

The herbal name of this mushroom, Pleurotusostreatus or P. sapidus, originates from the word for the lining of the thorax that covers the lungs, pleura, and is family to our word for the aggravation of that lining, pleurisy. All things considered; the state of the mushroom suggested this name. Ostreatus is Latin for "shellfish," and sapidus means "tasty" or "sapid."

Description, Habitat, and Season

Shellfish mushrooms grow from spring to fall on the sides of biting the dust hardwood trees or from the tops or sides of dead stumps, and they are adjusted down at the edges, with topsy turvy thick, intense stalks and white gills, caps of inconsistent size, and a fragile smell like clams. Pleurotus is frequently accessible in supermarkets, as it is currently grown industrially.

{ Recipes }

At the point when you find clam mushrooms, slice off just the fresh parts of the bargain's tops or the small young growth. The old part nearest to the stalks might be extreme. Pleurotus need conscientious cleaning to expel the little hard dark creepy crawlies that like to live in the gills. Absorb them warm salted water for a couple of moments, jar them here and there in the water, and drain and pat them dry before utilizing. Sliced, sautéed, and made into soup or a goulash, they are particularly awesome, and they taste a lot of like scalloped clams.

Boletus

Boletes (Boletus castaneus) are great top choices in Europe and picking up ubiquity in America. In Italy these dearest fungi are called porcini ("pig nourishment"), in France, cèpes (this word gets from an Old French word for onion, caepa), and in Germany, Steinpilz, or "stone mushrooms." (They may in fact show up from a separation like stones.) The genus name Boletus originates from bolo, the word for "ball," and the species name, castaneus, Latin for "chestnut," presumably alludes to their toasty brown color. They are likewise called B. edulis, the "edible boletus."

Description, Habitat, and Season

Boletes are large fall mushrooms, three crawls to a foot across, and grow in coniferous forests in America and Europe. They have brown, dry, adjusted tops with velvety pores underneath instead of gills and fat reticulated (crisscrossed like netting) stalks. Having tried most likely two dozen distinct boletes, the chestnut, or edible, boletus is the just a single I would prescribe. Some are poisonous: Avoid any that are red or that stain blue when a bit of the tissue is severed. The American chestnut boletus sees alike that is generous, however unpleasant tasting. The ones you need are toasty brown, and have firm ivory tissue, a gentle earthy scent, and a wonderful taste. History and Lore Boletes are brilliant, and safe if you distinguish them cautiously. They obviously dry well, and that is the means by which they are sold in Italy despite the fact that the ones I've attempted in Virginia have formed before I could dry them out. Boletes are frequently the "toadstools" you find in representations for fantasies; mythical people are supposed to use the big boleti for resting places.

{ Recipes }

Porcini in Puff Pastry (Serves four to six.) Preheat the oven to 400°F. Defrost 1 sheet of business puff baked good for 20 minutes and fold it into a 12" x 14" square shape. Sauté 1 cup or so sliced boletus (or other) mushrooms in 2 Tbsp. margarine with 1 or 2 squashed or minced cloves garlic, and season to taste with salt, pepper, a press of lemon juice, and a dispersing of nutmeg. Sprinkle the lightly browned fungi with 2 Tbsp. flour and mix until a roux is formed. Add 2 to 4 Tbsp. overwhelming cream to the mix, mixing great. The sauce ought to be thick. Spoon the mix down the focal point of the turned-out mixture, overlap the two sides over the center, and press a fork along the two closures to seal the puff. Rapidly brush the top with cream before placing it in the oven, to upgrade browning. Prepare 15 to 20 minutes, or until puffed and brilliant. Let cool around 10 minutes. Slice for a superb first course.

Coprinus

Coprinopsisatramentarius and Coprinellusmicaceus, both called inky caps, are modest in the world of fungi. The genus name originates from the Greek word kopros, signifying "fertilizer." They regularly grow where there is deadwood, or in fields frequented by dairy animals. The C. micaceus has granules much like the tops of sugar treats (mica in Latin is "piece" or "grain"), while C. atramentarius (which means just "edible") doesn't; else they are similar. The largest of the autodigestive genus, Coprinuscomatus, the shaggymane mushroom, has scales that become wavy or shaggy, and gills that become inky with age. Extreme lethargies are the Latin word for "hair." Shaggymanes can be found along cleared roadways, driveways, and walkways, just as in fields and lawns.

Description, Habitat, and Season

The coprini are bell-shaped mushrooms for the most part on thin, fragile stalks, regularly found in urban settings, particularly around the stumps or bases of old spoiling trees, and sometimes they are as thick as a rug. You can find them in spring, summer, and harvest time, in damp weather after rain. They are grayish brown, profoundly striated, packed together, and recognizable because they are autodigestive. That means that the old specimens have a wet, dark, dissolved appearance at the edges, caused by the procedure of self-processing. They run in size from under an inch to about two inches in diameter. Coprini might be disregarded by some because a significant number of them are small and difficult to clean: They push dirt up with them, on top of them, and are packed so thickly that it's sometimes difficult to get them to leave their hunks of dirt. They are additionally thin-fleshed and break no problem at all. However, all the coprini are completely scrumptious, and to my mind, worth the difficulty. Likewise, you don't need to go far to find them. They most likely grow some place on your street, or in your yard, or close to your woodpile. They love the mulched ground underneath our azaleas. I've seen them come up through solid driveways and, once, next to a bathroom toilet, during a rainy summer. I have as of late read that the coprini's autodigestive rule shields your liver from handling alcohol; along these lines you should not to drink alcohol within a few hours of eating coprini, nor eat them within a few hours of drinking alcohol.

{ Recipes }

Sautéed Coprini (For rice, pizza, or pasta.)

Wash coprini cautiously, disposing of any old, weakening specimens. Drain them completely on a lot of paper towels or kitchen towels. Liquefy 3 or 4 Tbsp. margarine or olive oil over medium heat and add the drained mushrooms. Season with somewhat salt and pepper, some garlic if you like, and a crush of lemon juice. Being thin fleshed, the coprini cook down rapidly and discharge a dark, rich sauce. Now, you can dry them out by keeping them over the heat until the fluid is evaporated and use them to scatteron pizza. Or then again you can add a little cream to the mushrooms before they dry out and serve them on rice or pasta.

Field Mushrooms

The field mushroom, Agaricuscampestris, is America's most famous mushroom. Its nearby family member, A. bisporus, or the doublesporedAgaricus, is the catch mushroom accessible fresh in grocery stores and the mushroom found in financially canned mushroom soup. A large relative is the portobello, found fresh nowadays in grocery stores. They are the fungi most widely used in America, and are called, simply, mushrooms. Agaricus originates from a word in Latin, ager, related to "section of land" and "agriculture," signifying "gainful field" or "field." Campestris is related to "grounds" in English, and in

Latin it, as well, means "plain," "open level spot," or "field." Both names advise unmistakably where this mushroom is to be found. The French name, champignon (champs in addition to pignon), means "field nut."

Description, Habitat, and Season

The most loved habitats of field mushrooms are fairways, fields where steers munch, parks, and wide lawns. They like wet weather and grow in pre-fall or late summer, sometimes in prodigious quantities, frequently in small or large circles, from white buttons about an inch in diameter to big specimens five inches across. Their color is whitish to pale beige. The way to distinguish them is to pick a young, an old, and an in the middle of example. The young buttons have tender, pale pink or tissue colored gills, sometimes still collapsed into themselves; in time the young gills darken to a chocolatey brown, and the old, larger specimens have dark rosy brown or blackish brown gills. Maintain a strategic distance from any field mushrooms with white gills. Bring a flat-bottomed basket to accumulate field mushrooms, for they are somewhat fragile and have a slight tendency to break. Additionally, bring a blade, with which to cut the caps off just beneath the caps. This keeps away from a large portion of the dirt that so regularly sticks to the stems, which are stringy and intense anyway.

{ Recipes }

Attempt to get over the dirt field mushrooms, at that point wash them off with water instead of dousing them, for they smudge up water like wipes and you may wind up with a watery wreckage of spore stained mushrooms. In the event that you need to dunk them, at that point drain them completely on paper towels or kitchen towels before you cook them. In the late-summer, field mushrooms are frequently so various you can accumulate a year's stock in 60 minutes. Subsequent to sautéing them in butter, you can freeze them in small containers for year-round use.

Shiitake

I had never known about the shiitake mushroom (Lentinula edodes) when this book previously showed up in the nineties. There's an explanation behind that: These famous fungi are genuinely late appearances to this country. My companion Ann Tutwiler Rogers Carman reveals to me that shiitake means "oak mushroom" in Japanese (shii is "oak tree"; take means "mushroom"). These fungi grow wild on different species ofoak (and sometimes other) trees in their local Asian forests, yet no one but once in a while can be found in the wild right now, their rate grows as time passes. They are a decaying fungus (which says their raison d'être is to break down oak wood). Their gleaming spores coast around in Asian forests and land on oak branches. (Or then again, a shiitake is placed upon an oak branch.) The spores "eat" the wood until the branch spoils enough to fall to the ground. The shock of the fall "awakens" the lethargic mushrooms, driving them to fruit. So, shiitake growers, who taint oak logs with spores, regularly drop their logs to the ground with an end goal to stun them into growing. They additionally frequently absorb the logs water to saturate them and make them fruit. Shiitake are believed to cherish tempests, and a few growers really play hints of roar to their harvests and blaze light around them to mimic lightning.

Description, Habitat, and Season

Shiitake are brown with whitish gills, three to ten inches across, with a leathery texture and woody stems. They grow gregariously on oak logs. Shiitake (solitary and plural are the equivalent) are mushrooms that are flavorfully edible, yet additionally medicinally useful, as they are antiviral and antibacterial. They are useful in stifling herpes episodes, and tests have found them promising as treatments for hypersensitivities, joint pain, and even melanomas. This makes them wholesome powerhouses. They're likewise expected to be capably Spanish fly, particularly the ones with broke tops. They grow all through the warm months, and sometimes, after a good splashing, on warm days in the winter.

History and Lore

Shiitake are charmingly human. They are said to kick the bucket whenever left without anyone else, however, to thrive in the company of their kindred shiitake and in the company of individuals. In Asia they are viewed as an image of long life and health. In any case, right now shiitake was confused with another Asian mushroom, and it was long believed that shiitake would colonize on and pulverize all the scaffolds and railroad ties made of chestnut oak (Quercusprinus) or white oak (Quercus alba), its preferred host plants. Accordingly, it was prohibited right now the 1970s when the facts got fixed. In the mediating years, the shiitake has been grown locally in warm atmospheres all over the place, with some attendant wilding. I have a humble shiitake ranch in my garden behind some container shrubberies, and I put firewood logs close by quite a long while prior to check whether the shiitake would send a few spores to my fire logs. Mine didn't produce mushrooms, however my companion Milt McGrady dumped a heap of firewood close to his shiitake logs, and after two years shiitake developed there, therefore demonstrating that wild shiitake exist. The spores, he says, must fall on ideal substrate to produce fungi—typically just certain oaks, yet maybe periodically, he thinks, on other oak trees, as well.

{ Recipes }

Shiitake are used fresh and dried and are flavorful sautéed in butter and served over wild rice. The stems are woody, so they ought to be evacuated. If the fungi are dried, they should be reconstituted in warm water before cooking. Once reconstituted, they might be used as some other mushroom. Shiitake have a pleasant chewy consistency and a smoky, meaty flavor, and they do well with moderate cooking.

Signs and Symptoms of Substance Abuse-Overdose Assistance

Remember your motivation for attempting to find out if somebody is doing alcohol and additionally drugs-To Identify and Help as opposed to Catch and Punish.

General: General and explicit guides to detection of alcohol and drug use, and definition of addiction.

Contents:

    I.   General Guide to Detection
    II.   Definition of Addiction
    III. Pupil Dilation
    IV.   Signs and Symptoms
    V.   Paraphernalia a) S/S Chart Version
    VI.   Drug Facts
    VII. Articles and Other Resources
    VIII. Drug Pictures/Resources
    IX.   Topics
    X.   Additional Articles (Alcoholism, Drugs, Teenage Addiction, Interventions)
    XI.   Overdose and Emergency Intervention Techniques

I. Explicit: General Guide to Detection

Unexpected changes in work or school attendance, nature of work, work yield, grades, discipline.

Uncommon flare-ups or flare-ups of emotion. Withdrawal from obligation. General changes in by and large demeanor. Crumbling of physical appearance and grooming.

Wearing of shades at improper times. Ceaseless wearing of long-sleeved articles of clothing especially in sweltering weather or hesitance to wear short sleeved clothing when suitable. Relationship with known substance abusers. Strange obtaining of cash from companions, associates or guardians. Stealing small things from boss, home or school. Clandestine behavior with respect to activities and possessions; ineffectively hid endeavors to keep away from consideration and doubt, for example, frequent trips to extra spaces, restroom, storm cellar, and so forth.

II. Specific: DSM-IV Definition of Addiction

A maladaptive example of substance use, prompting clinically critical debilitation or pain, as manifested by (at least three) of the accompanying, occurring whenever in a similar year time frame:

1) Tolerance, as characterized by both of the accompanying:

    a. A requirement for notably expanded measures of the substance to accomplish intoxication or wanted effect.

    b. Notably lessened effect with continued use of a similar measure of the substance.

2) Withdrawal, as manifested by both of the accompanying:

    a. The trademark withdrawal disorder for the substance.

    b. The equivalent (or a firmly related) substance is taken to soothe or stay away from withdrawal symptoms.

3) The substance is regularly taken in larger sums or over a longer period than was intended (loss of control).

4) There is a persevering want or fruitless endeavors to chop down or control substance use (loss of control).

5) A great arrangement of time is spent on activities important to get the substance, use the substance, or recuperate from its effects (preoccupation).

6) Important social, occupational, or recreational activities are surrendered or reduced because of substance use (continuation regardless of adverse consequences).

7) The substance use is continued regardless of information on having a tireless or repetitive physical or mental issue that is likely to have been caused or exacerbated by the substance (adverse consequences).

III. Specific: Pupil Dilation

Before you do anything, think about this. There are two trains of thought before detection and intervention. One thought is to get and rebuff, and the other is to recognize and help-remember why you are doing this, and the intervention will turn out to be much better.

Note: A 6mm, 7mm, or 8mm pupil size could show that a person is affected by cocaine, crack, and meth, hallucinogens, precious stone, bliss, or another stimulant. A 1mm or 2mm pupil size could demonstrate a person affected by heroin, sedatives, or another depressant. A pupil near pinpoint could demonstrate use. A pupil totally dilated could demonstrate use. Smothered wide pupils are indicative of crack, methamphetamine, cocaine, and stimulant use. Pinpoint pupils are indicative of heroin, sedative, depressant use.

Different causes of pupil dilation

IV. Specific: Signs and Symptoms

Alcohol: Odor on the breath. Intoxication. Difficulty centering: coated appearance of the eyes. Uniquely detached behavior; or contentious and factious behavior. Slow (or unexpected in teenagers) weakening in personal appearance and cleanliness. Slow improvement of brokenness, particularly in work performance or schoolwork. Truancy (especially on Monday). Unexplained wounds and mishaps. Irritability. Flushed skin. Loss of memory (blackouts). Availability and utilization of alcohol turns into the focal point of social or expert activities. Changes in peer-bunch affiliations and companionships. Debilitated interpersonal connections (grieved marriage, unexplainable termination of profound connections, distance from close relatives).

Marijuana/Pot: Rapid, uproarious talking and explosions of chuckling straightly stages of intoxication. Sluggish or daze in the later stages. Absent mindedness in conversation. Aggravation in whites of eyes; pupils unlikely to be dilated. Smell similar to consumed rope on clothing or breath. Tendency to drive gradually - underneath speed limit. Contorted sense of time section - tendency to overestimate time interims. Use or possession of paraphernalia including insect cut, packs of moving papers, funnels or bongs. Marijuana users are difficult to perceive except if they are affected by the drug at the time of perception. Easygoing users may show none of the general symptoms. Marijuana has an unmistakable scent and might be a similar color or somewhat greener than tobacco.

Cocaine/Crack/Methamphetamines/Stimulants:
Extremely dilated pupils. Dry mouth and nose, terrible breath, frequent lip licking. Over the top activity, difficulty sitting despite everything, lack of enthusiasm for nourishment or rest. Crabby, pugnacious, apprehensive. Garrulous, however conversation regularly lacks congruity; changes subjects quickly. Runny nose, cold or constant sinus/nasal problems, nose drains. Use paraphernalia including small spoons, disposable cutters, reflect, little containers of white powder and plastic, glass or metal straws.

Depressants: Symptoms of alcohol intoxication without alcohol smell on breath (remember that depressants are frequently used with alcohol). Lack of outward appearance or activity. Flat effect. Limp appearance. Slurred speech. Note:

There are scarcely any readily apparent symptoms. Abuse might be shown by activities, for example, frequent visits to various physicians for prescriptions to treat" apprehension", "anxiety"," stress", and so forth.

Opiates/Prescription Drugs/Opium/Heroin/Codeine/Oxycontin

Lethargy, drowsiness. Choked pupils neglect to react to light. Redness and raw nostrils from breathing in heroin in power form. Scars (tracks) on internal arms or different parts of body, from needle infusions. Use or possession of paraphernalia, including syringes, bowed spoons, bottle caps, eyedroppers, elastic tubing, cotton and needles. Slurred speech. While there might be no readily apparent symptoms of pain-relieving abuse, it might be shown by frequent visits to various physicians or dental specialists for prescriptions to treat agony of vague birthplace. In cases where patient has incessant agony and abuse of drug is suspected, it might be shown by sums and recurrence taken.

Inhalants: Substance smell on breath and garments. Runny nose. Watering eyes. Drowsiness or obviousness. Poor muscle control. Lean towards bunch activity to being separated from everyone else. Presence of packs or clothes containing dry plastic concrete or other dissolvable at home, in storage at school or at work. Disposed of whipped cream, spray paint or similar chargers (users of nitrous oxide). Small containers named" incense" (users of butyl nitrite).

Solvents, Aerosols, Glue, Petrol: Nitrous Oxide - giggling gas, whippets, nitrous. Amyl Nitrate - snappers, poppers, pearlers, rushamie, Butyl Nitrate - storage space, jolt, shot, surge, peak, red gold. Slurred speech, weakened coordination, nausea, heaving, eased back breathing. Brain harm, torments in the chest, muscles, joints, heart inconvenience, extreme depression, weariness, loss of craving, bronchial fit, injuries on nose or mouth, nosebleeds, the runs, odd or crazy behavior, abrupt death, suffocation.

LSD/Hallucinogens: Extremely dilated pupils, (see note beneath). Warm skin, inordinate sweat and body scent. Contorted sense of sight, hearing, contacts; misshaped picture of self and time perception. Mood and behavior changes, the degree depending on passionate condition of the user and natural conditions Unpredictable flashback scenes even long after withdrawal (in spite of the fact that these are uncommon). Hallucinogenic drugs, which exist both naturally and in synthetic form, mutilate or upset tangible information, sometimes to a great degree. Hallucinogens occur naturally in essentially two forms, (peyote) cactus and psilocybin mushrooms.

A few chemical assortments have been synthesized, most strikingly, MDA, STP, and PCP. Hallucinogen utilization arrived at a topping the United States in the late 1960's, however declined presently because of a more extensive attention to the detrimental effects of use. However, an upsetting pattern showing resurgence in hallucinogen use by secondary school and school age persons across the nation has been recognized by law requirement. Except for PCP, all hallucinogens appear to share basic effects of use. Any bit of tangible perceptions might be modified to shifting degrees. Synesthesia, or the "seeing" of sounds, and the "hearing" of colors, is a typical symptom of hallucinogen use. Depersonalization, intense anxiety, and intense depression bringing about suicide have likewise been noted because of hallucinogen use. Note: there are a few forms of hallucinogens that are viewed as killjoys and choke pupil diameters.

PCP: Unpredictable behavior; mood may swing from resignation to violence for no apparent explanation. Symptoms of intoxication. Confusion; tumult and violence whenever presented to over the top tactile incitement. Dread, fear. Inflexible muscles. Peculiar stride. Stifled tangible perception (may experience severe wounds while showing up not to take note). Pupils may show up dilated. Veil like facial appearance. Drifting pupils seem to follow a moving article. Insensible (lethargic) if large sum consumed. Eyes might be open or shut.

Ecstasy: Confusion, depression, migraines, unsteadiness (from hangover/delayed consequences), muscle strain, alarm attacks, paranoia, possession of pacifiers (used to stop jaw grasping), candies, treats pieces of jewelry, mentholated medicated ointment, severe anxiety, sore jaw (from gripping teeth eventual outcomes), spewing or nausea (from hangover/eventual outcomes).

Signs that your teenager could be high on Ecstasy: Blurred vision, fast eye development, pupil dilation, chills or sweating, high body temperature, sweating profusely, dehydrated, confusion, faintness, paranoia or severe anxiety, stupor like state, transfixed on destinations and sounds, oblivious grasping of the jaw, pounding teeth, extremely tender.

V. DRUG SIGNS and SYMPTOMS

Stimulants (Cocaine, Ecstasy, Meth., Crystal)

Depressants (Heroin, Marijuana, Downers)

Hallucinogens (LSD)

Narcotics (Rx. Meds)

Inhalants (Paint, Gasoline, White Out)

PCP

Alcohol

Note: Paraphernalia-Keep in mind, that you may not find drugs, if you are looking for them, however you can as a rule find the paraphernalia related with use.

VI. Specific: Drug Facts

Incorporates identifiers, definitions, language of users and sellers. Drug Terms Slang and Street Terms.

VII. Specific: Other Resources and Articles

This the additional information for brain chemistry and the drug user).

VIII. Specific: Drug Pictures/Resources from the DEA

CHEMICAL CONTROL

Prologue TO DRUG CLASSES

Narcotics of Natural Origin

Opium, Morphine, Codeine, Thebaine

Semi-Synthetic Narcotics

Heroin Hydromorphone Oxycodone Hydrododone

Synthetic Narcotics

Meperidine

Narcotics Treatment Drugs

Methadone Dextroproxyphene Fentanyl PentazocineButorphanol

DEPRESSANTS Barbiturates

Controlled Substances Uses and Effects (Chart) Benzodiazepines Gamma

HydroxybutricAcidParaldehyde, Chloral HydrateGlutethimide 7

MethaqualoneMeprobamate

Recently Marketed Drugs

STIMULANTS Cocaine Amphetamines

Methcathinone, Methylphenidate

ANORECTIC DRUGS cap

CANNABIS Marijuana Hashish Oil

HALLUCINOGENS LSD Psilocybin & Psilocybin and Other Tryptamines Peyote and Mescaline MDMA (Ecstasy) and Other Phenethylamines Phencyclidine (PCP) and Related Drugs Ketamine

STEROIDS

INHALANTS

IX. Specific: NICD Topics

Do you have questions relating to addiction/addictions/substance abuse? Family Resources for the family, intervention information, support, and directing. Clinical information, specialist and pros index, terminology and lexicon of terms.

Treatment.

The Villa at Scottsdale-Providing a full continuum of care for the treatment of alcoholism and drug addiction.

Alcohol and Drug Addiction Survival Kit

General: A series, for the individual, family, companions, managers, teachers, experts, and so on prevention, intervention, treatment, recuperation, backslide prevention, support, and different issues relating to alcoholism and drug addiction.

1. Prevention-Includes tips on the best way to converse with your children about alcohol, tobacco, and drugs.

2. Detection of Signs and Symptoms-A guide to detection of alcohol and different drug utilization.

3. Definition of Addiction-A DSM-IV definition of precisely what establishes alcoholism and drug addiction.

4. Intervention-Interventions can and accomplish work. We will tell you the best way to do it effectively.

5. Treatment and Housing-A treatment place and halfway house locator.

6. Support-Some guides to how to support somebody while they are in treatment.

7. After Care-What to do before and after discharge from treatment.

8. Recuperation/Relapse Prevention-Addiction can surface once more, as backslide.

9. Different Issues-Issues to think about with respect to those influenced by substance abuse, just as everyone around them.

10. References-A rundown of the individuals who contributed to this series of articles.

Articles Medical Today Dr. William Gallagher walks us through his use of DNFT with his patients. Psychotherapy Today Psychologist Jim Maclaine stays up with the latest with his articles of understanding, treatment, and healing. Directing Today Therapist Thom Rutledge gives a creative approach to dealing with life on life's standing through his interesting advising meetings. Big Book Bytes Author Shelly Marshall shares by means of the Big Book on issues of worry to those in recovery. All pages are set-up to copy, for use by guides, experts, patrons, and others.

Recovery Today Interviews of people in recovery, about drug abuse, addictions, alcoholism, recovery, restraint, spirituality, wisdom, experience, quality, and hope. Tune in month to month for new articles!

A.A. History Author Dick B. will return you to a time when the recovery rates were as high as 93%.

Journaling Today A series of informative articles by Author Doreene Clementon how, why, and what to expound on.

Spirituality Today Author Carol Tuttle takes us higher than ever on our spiritual excursion.

Articles of God and Faith Features 100's of topics relating to God, confidence, spirituality, and the sky is the limit from there.

Life Today Everyday life experiences from people everywhere throughout the world. Life, Addictions, Recovery, Hope, Inspiration, Wisdom, Advice, thus substantially more. Tune in all the time to perceive what others have and are experiencing. Find hope from the experiences of others.

Steps Today Recovery Peer and Advisory Board Member Dean G. gives creative approach to dealing with life on life's standing by means of his exceptional recovery meetings.

Step Work/Relapse Prevention This administration is intended to assist with step work, with statements and pages from the Big Book, with forms prepared to copy and use. There is a segment committed to backslide prevention too.

X. Specific: Additional Articles

Health and Medical News, recordings, content from the world of medicine, health, and clinical.

Ecstasy information.

How Do I Converse with My Kids About Alcohol?

How Do I converse with my kids about drugs?

How Do I talk with my teenager about alcohol and drugs?

What does a crack channel resemble?

Family assistance for substance abuse.

Addiction treatment for my teenager.

Overdose or OD Information

XI. Specific: Overdose and Emergency Intervention Techniques

Drug Overdose-Drug overdoses can be incidental or deliberately. The measure of a drug expected to cause an overdose differs with the type of drug and the person taking it. Overdoses from prescription or over the counter (OTC) medicines, "street" drugs, as well as alcohol can be life threatening. Know that mixing certain medications or "street" drugs with alcohol can likewise execute.

Physical symptoms of a drug overdose change with the type of drug(s) taken. They include: Abnormal breathing Slurred speech Lack of coordination Slow or quick pulse Low or raised body temperature Enlarged or small eye pupils Reddish face Heavy sweating Drowsiness Violent upheavals Delusions or potentially hallucinations Unconsciousness which may prompt trance like state (Note: A diabetic who takes insulin may show a portion of the above symptoms in the event that the person in question is having an insulin reaction.)

Parents need to look for signs of illegal drug and alcohol use in their children. Morning hangovers, the smell of alcohol, and red streaks in the whites of the eyes are clear signs of alcohol use. Things, for example, pipes, moving papers, eye droppers and butane lighters might be the primary telling signs that somebody is mishandling drugs. Another hint is behavior changes, for example, Lack of craving Insomnia, Hostility Mental, Confusion, Depression Mood Swings, Secretive Behavior, Social Segregation, Deep Rest, Hallucinations.

Prevention-Accidental prescription and over-the-counter medication overdoses might be prevented by asking your doctor or drug specialist: What is the medication and for what reason is it being prescribed? How and when should the medication be taken and for to what extent? (Follow the instructions precisely as given.) Can the medication be taken with different medicines or alcohol or not? Are there any foods to keep away from while taking this medication? What are the conceivable reactions? What are the signs of an overdose and what ought to be done if it occurs? Should any activities be kept away from, for example, sitting in the sun, working overwhelming apparatus, driving? Should the medicine despite everything be taken if there is a prior ailment?

To maintain a strategic distance from medication overdoses: Never take a medicine prescribed for another person. Never give or take medication in the dark. Prior to each dose, always read the name on the jug to be sure it is the right medication. Always tell the doctor of any past symptoms or adverse reactions to medication just as new and bizarre symptoms that occur subsequent to taking the medicine. Always store medications in bottles with childproof tops and place those bottles on high retires, out of a child's compass, or in bolted cupboards. Take the prescribed dose, not more. Keep medications in their unique containers to debilitate unlawful drug use among children: Set a good model for your children by not utilizing drugs yourself. Teach your child to state "NO" to drugs and alcohol. Clarify the threats of drug use, including the risk of AIDS. Find a workable pace children's companions and their parents. Know where your children are and whom they are with. Tune in to your children and help them to communicate their feelings and fears. Urge your children to participate in healthy activities, for example, sports, exploring, network-based youth projects and humanitarian effort. Figure out how to perceive the signs of drug and alcohol abuse.

Inquiries to Pose:

Is the person not breathing and has no pulse? Medical aid Perform Cyprinids the person not breathing, however has a pulse? Emergency treatment Perform Rescue Breathing AND is the person oblivious? Medical aid lay the victim down on their left side and check airway, breathing and pulse regularly before emergency care. Perform mouth to mouth or Rescue Breathing varying. And does the person have any of these signs?

Hallucinations Confusion Convulsions Breathing moderate and shallow as well as slurring their words

Do you speculate the person has taken an overdose of drugs? Emergency treatment Call Poison Control Center. Follow the Poison Control Center's instructions. Approach the victim serenely and carefully. Walk the person around to keep that person alert and to help the syrup of ipecac work quicker, in the event that you were advised to give this to the victim. Likewise, see "Poisoning". Also, is the person's personality out of nowhere hostile, vicious and forceful? Emergency treatment Use alert. Ensure yourself. Try not to turn your back to the victim or move unexpectedly before the person in question. If you can, see that the victim doesn't hurt you, oneself. Remember, the victim is affected by a drug. Call the police to assist you in the event that you can't handle the circumstance. Leave and find a protected place to stay until the police show up. Also, have you or another person inadvertently taken more than the prescribed dose of a prescription or over-the-counter medication? Try not to perform any strategy except if it involves life and death! If you are uncertain of what you are doing, if it's not too much trouble follow the instructions given by a 911 administrator.

Conclusion

You can't always predict the effects of magic mushrooms until the medication has already been taken. Unfortunately, the effects of magic mushrooms are unreliable and unpredictable as with most hallucinogenic drugs. Many users may experience a high spiritual or otherwise enlightening while others may experience an "evil" trip that could lead to extreme fear, anxiety, depression or schizophrenia such as outbursts and chaos. The effects of psilocybin are mostly short lived. The medication appears to wear off after a few hours, and no significant side effects for the patient are known. Unfortunately this does not mean that it is safe or openly accepted to take magic mushrooms to get high. There is a risk of toxicity, and it may be harmful to use these mushrooms, despite the lack of long-term side effects following drug use.

The controversial area of research is the use of psilocybin, a chemical which occurs naturally in some mushrooms. Psilocybin has been shown to be effective in treating alcohol and cigarette addiction. New studies show that anxiety and depression in some cancer patients may be eased by the hallucinogenic medication. Several reports have documented mood raising effects that lasted at least several weeks after eating the fungus. While fungus has intrigued people for a long time, it may finally come into a new era where its healing properties and unknown qualities are being discovered. The mushroom could very well hold the key to some long-established mysteries and diseases. For thousands of years, medical use of mushrooms has been going on with good reason: they are effective. It is time for more focused work to explore more uses and forces of this delicate nature gift.

[Page intentionally left blank]

PSILOCYBIN GROWING BIBLE

The Complete Psilocybin Mushroom Cultivation Guide Step by Step to Grow Indoor and Outdoor Your Magic Psychedelic Mushrooms with Safety Measure.

By Tyler Barrett

© Copyright 2020 by Tyler Barrett

All rights reserved.

This document is geared towards providing exact and reliable information with regards to the topic and issue covered. The publication is sold with the idea that the publisher is not required to render accounting, officially permitted, or otherwise, qualified services. If advice is necessary, legal or professional, a practiced individual in the profession should be ordered.

- From a Declaration of Principles which was accepted and approved equally by a Committee of the American Bar Association and a Committee of Publishers and Associations.

In no way is it legal to reproduce, duplicate, or transmit any part of this document in either electronic means or in printed format. Recording of this publication is strictly prohibited and any storage of this document is not allowed unless with written permission from the publisher. All rights reserved.

The information provided herein is stated to be truthful and consistent, in that any liability, in terms of inattention or otherwise, by any usage or abuse of any policies, processes, or directions contained within is the solitary and utter responsibility of the recipient reader. Under no circumstances will any legal responsibility or blame be held against the publisher for any reparation, damages, or monetary loss due to the information herein, either directly or indirectly.

Respective authors own all copyrights not held by the publisher.

The information herein is offered for informational purposes solely, and is universal as so. The presentation of the information is without contract or any type of guarantee assurance.

The trademarks that are used are without any consent, and the publication of the trademark is without permission or backing by the trademark owner. All trademarks and brands within this book are for clarifying purposes only and are the owned by the owners themselves, not affiliated with this document.

Disclaimer

All Erudition contained in this book is given for informational and educational purposes only. The author is not in any way accountable for any results or outcomes that emanate from using this material. Constructive attempts have been made to provide information that is both accurate and effective, but the author is not bound for the accuracy or use/misuse of information.

Foreword

First, I will like to thank you for taking the first step of trusting me and deciding to purchase/read this life transforming eBook. Thanks for spending your time and resources on this material. I can assure you of exact blueprint I lay bare in the information manual you are currently reading. It has transformed lives, and I strongly believe it will equally transform your life too. All the information I presented in this Do-It-Yourself is easy to digest and practice.

Contents

CHAPTER 1 135

CHAPTER 2 137

CHAPTER 3 142

CHAPTER 4 159

CHAPTER 5 170

CHAPTER 6 187

CHAPTER 7 191

CHAPTER 8 199

CHAPTER 9 206

CHAPTER 10 210

CHAPTER 11 215

CHAPTER 12 222

CHAPTER 13 236

CHAPTER 1
Where to grow your mushroom

Outdoor cultivation

Growing outdoor mushrooms are ideal in many ways because the forest (or any dreary area with good humidity and air flow) provides the perfect fruiting conditions without the need of the farmer for any climate control. In fact, the forest is where the mushrooms we grow come from, so why not just grow them out there? This is the thought which led to the development of Cornell's initial mushroom research and extension project led by Professor Kenneth Mudge (now Emeritus), who was particularly interested in agroforestry, or the combination of trees, forests, and crop production.

Ken has been studying many species for nearly 15 years, mainly concentrating on log-grown shiitake mushrooms as they quickly proved to have the most economical viability. We also know that mane, oyster, wine cap Stropharia can be successfully grown outdoors, and a few other minor species. The main restriction with outdoor or forest cultivation is that only the log-grown shiitake can grow consistently enough out of the species mentioned above to produce weekly mushrooms, a necessary part of the supply chain to a farm company. This is due to the unique property that shiitake logs can be soaked or "forced" into fruit by immersing the logs in water for 12-24 hours, which encourages them to bear fruit. This process can be used to grow relatively consistently mushrooms from around the first week of June through the middle to late part of October, at least in Central New York's climate. Although efficient, the other species produce fruit on their own, and so are not good choices if the goal is to yield consistent market yields.

Indoor Growing

Once we step out of the woods and into an enclosed space, the list of species that we can reliably grow begins to expand considerably. In addition, we must also begin to monitor and maintain the ideal environment for the different production stages, from incubation to fruiting. And probably the most challenging thing, we need to take extra measures to reduce and eliminate contamination sources in our substrates, which will arrest and prevent fruiting of our desired mushrooms. With outdoor production, this issue is almost non-existent, a big advantage point. Indoor farming systems are sometimes called "controlled agricultural environment," which includes other systems such as hydroponics, aquaponics, and greenhouse production. Unlike CEA systems used for greens and herbs, mushrooms can be produced in locations with limited infrastructure and resources for production start-up and sustainability. However, considerations and controls need to be made regarding the present temperature, humidity, light, and airflow.

A major advantage of indoor manufacturing is that systems can be adapted to work in a wide range of abandoned and underused farm infrastructure including barns, outbuildings, high tunnels, and storage. The basements, shipping containers and warehouse spaces can easily be retrofitted for production in an urban environment. This positions mushrooms as a system accessible for both rural and urban farms, as well as those farmers with limited capital and access to other start-up resources.

CHAPTER 2
Sterile culture technique

Mushroom food (properly known as its substratum) is much like human food: a nutritious mixture that contains a balance of carbohydrates, proteins, minerals, and vitamins. Like our food too, I find a variety of microorganisms quite delightful, as a loaf of bread left out in the kitchen counter will quickly prove for more than a few days. Unlike humans, however, fungi are also micro-organisms and must compete with any other neighborhood micro-organisms for food. Bacteria and molds have a competitive edge because they can reproduce thousands, even millions of times faster than the average species of mushrooms can. Any substrate that even contains a single mold spore or bacterium will likely end up a moldy or mushy mess. Furthermore, in the average room, the average cubic centimeter of air contains more than 100,000 particles. No matter how scrupulously clean you think it is, an invisible, silent rain of mold spores, dust particles, and pollen grains settles constantly on every horizontal surface in your home. The only way to prevent these critics from hijacking the mushroom cultures is to ensure that they never get on to them first. There are two general ways to do this: by working in a truly clean (i.e., sterile) environment, they thoroughly kill whatever molds or bacteria are there, to begin with, and exclude any other. We extract pollutants from our products by sterilizing them in a pressure cooker, where practically no living thing may withstand the high temperatures (1210 C/ 255' F) and pressures (15 psi) within them. We then create a sterile working environment by filtering the air in our workspace and/or using chemical disinfectants to sterilize it.

Those two techniques constitute the technique of sterile or aseptic farming, which is by far the most important thing you need to know to succeed in cultivating the mushrooms. Let me reiterate this for emphasis: The most important thing you can learn from this book is the sterile culture technique. If you do not figure out this one, none of the methods of cultivation will work, no matter how closely you follow the instructions. If you're really, really lucky, you might harvest one or two mushrooms, but mostly you'll have a gleaming array of blue, green, and black molds and a slimy, stinky bacteria collection. Many would-be mushroom growers have failed right here, and those who succeeded (including your humble authors) have learned the hard way of using sterile culture techniques and why. It is our hope that the strategies presented in this chapter will show you the easy way, saving you time and heartbreak.

Cleaning your work area

The preparation of a clean workspace is the first task. Ideally, you can only dedicate a room or space to your mushroom projects, like a spare bedroom or an unused walk-in closet. If there is no such space, then much of the laboratory work can be accomplished in an average kitchen, but this requires you to establish and maintain a pristine level of cleanliness. The kitchen competes with the bathroom as the house's messiest and biologically active room, and the counts of molds there tend to be very high. Working in a kitchen, on the other hand, provides convenient access to a water source and furnace top. If you're planning to devote a separate space to mushrooming, make sure it's near the kitchen. There's no point in sterilizing your materials just to carry them into your laboratory through a dirty house. A good-sized table should be in the workspace, preferably one with a continuous, easily cleaned upper surface. Formica or enamel is ideal because before each use you will need to wipe the workbench with alcohol. If you have a wooden table, consider putting on top of it a piece of thin plywood with a plastic laminate surface, or a piece of heavy, thick vinyl when working. Similarly, it should be easy to clean the workspace floor (linoleum or tile), and easy to inspect for cleanliness. Carpets are spores and dust repositories, millions of which are kicked into the air every step of the way and should be avoided if possible. The walls must be clean (a fresh coat of paint wouldn't hurt), and any other room spaces and surfaces should be cleaned thoroughly. Use a solution for disinfecting if practical (orange-oil based products are good as they are mild but effective biocides and environmentally friendly). Obviously, if you work in your kitchen, you can't disinfect every surface whenever you plan to use it, but you should still give it a regular deep cleaning and disinfect as much of it as you can before every use. Space should be void of drafts to minimize air circulation around your cultures. Windows should be tightly closed, heating or air-conditioning ducts should be covered, and doors should be closed long before you start work. Whenever possible eliminate other sources of contamination from the room. Potted plants, fish tanks, food plates for pets, litter boxes: get them all out of there. It is helpful to run an air-filtration device in the space too.

Good ones nowadays cost less than $100 and are silent and efficient enough to run continuously. Make sure the unit you are buying is rated HEF'A. HEPA stands for Particulate Air with high efficiency. It is an official filter rating which means it captures 0.1 microns (1/100th of a millimeter) and larger particles, or 99.97 percent of airborne solid matter. So, give the air in the room a thorough scrubbing, we keep our filter on low at all times and run it up for at least an hour before working in the lab. Finally, in your immediate work area, you need to clean the air. This can be done by working inside a glove box, an enclosed space that can be thoroughly disinfected and is draft-free, or in front of a flow hood, a large HEPA filter unit that blows a steady stream of pure sterile air over your workspace, excluding all contaminants. A glove box can be quickly and inexpensively installed but is less effective because the air from the space can find its way inside.

Personal Hygiene

Now that your space has been cleaned and prepared, it's time to consider the other primary source of contamination in your makeshift laboratory: you. Your hair, body, and clothes are an Amazon jungle of bacteria, viruses, and fungi that are all invisible to your eyes, mostly harmless to you or others, but deadly to the mushroom cultures. You should be as neat as possible before each work session to keep that nasty horde to a minimum. That means showering, drying off with a freshly laundered towel and dressing immediately before working in a clean set of clothes. It's also important to choose your clothing; don't wear long-sleeved shirts or loose-fitting items that might flop around while you work. If you've got long hair, tie it up on your head. Use isopropyl (rubbing) alcohol, wash your hands and lower arms and always wear disposable surgical gloves when operating (wipe the outside of the gloves too, use alcohol).

Mental Hygiene

Just as you've packed your workspace and body, make sure you're still taking care of your state of mind before working. Mental hygiene is as critical as personal hygiene because the way you work will be affected by your state of mind, and if you are disturbed or rushed, you are likely to make mistakes or contaminate your culture. Your laboratory movements should be systematic, calculated and deliberate. Avoid unnecessary fast or jerky movements, as they produce only unwanted air currents. Take your moment. If you're hurried, slow down or save the idea for a day you've got more time. In the same way, ask your partner, kids, dog or cat not to enter the room or interrupt you while you are working and disconnecting your phone. Play calming, elevating music if you like, but avoid Stockhausen or speed metal, unless you find it to your ears to relax.

CHAPTER 3

Equipment and supplies

Mushroom cultivation requires equipment, including many specific devices. A couple of these items are explicit to the point that they must be bought from mushroom cultivation supply houses, however, most can without much of a stretch be found at I an assortment of neighborhood sources. A significant number of the materials you need fire likewise sold for some other, increasingly mundane reason; while making shopping simpler, this has the additional advantage of giving good spread to those, wishing to stay under the radar on their cultivation activities. Home improvement shops, kitchen, and café supply houses, pet stores, home fermenting providers, and garden focuses are the fortune troves of the stealthy (or simply economical) mushroom cultivator. Whenever conceivable, we have attempted to give numerous general sources to every one of the items you may require.

Equipment

Pressure Cooker

This will be one of the most utilized items in your cultivation apparatus shed, so it is important to get a better than average one right from the start. Since you will use it to disinfect generally large items, and in quantity, size is basic. If you can manage the cost of a larger unit than you at first need, get it, since you will likely need to update later anyway. The key determinant for what size you ought to get is the number of quart jars you can securely clean at once. Since bricklayer jars are unpredictably shaped, generally few can fit easily inside even the largest pressure cooker, constraining the measure of material you can process at once. In this manner, we recommend getting a unit that can hold at least seven-quart jars without a moment's delay; the model we use, the All American #941, holds more than twice that many.

There are various options as to what brand and type to get, yet one stands apart from the group: The All-American brand, manufactured by the Aluminum Foundry of Wisconsin. All American pressure cookers are the best-made, generally reliable, and accessible to the safest. The company has been doing business for a long time, and since they were first introduced, the design of their pressure cookers has not fundamentally changed. They're made primarily of overwhelming test cast aluminum, and they don't have elastic seals or wear-out sections. Replacement parts are readily accessible, and even a 20-year-old unit purchased at a secondhand shop or on eBay can be made to work well as new.

Like smaller, lower-priced kitchen pressure cookers, all Americans have a huge, extremely accurate dial scale that lacks a method of determining the internal pressure decisively. They are also intended to hold a vacuum after cooling which is necessary to prevent the existence of non-sterile air in your crops.

There are two general types of pressure cookers to choose from: those with or similar to a vapor discharge valve, and those with a metal-weighted "rocker" that releases steam at any point above a certain pressure level. The last sort should be prevented, if possible, as this rapid arrival of pressure would cause the fluids inside the cooker to boil over, dramatically demolishing the media and wrecking. Pressure cookers can be used in rocker style, but they need increasingly rigorous monitoring during use to avoid these accidents. (Each American makes the two types; the type of stopcock they call pressure "sterilizers," while the weighted rockers are known as pressure "canners.") Whatever brand and model of pressure cooker you choose, make sure it's in good working order and you understand its operation and well-being (i.e., read the manual). Make sure all seals and gaskets match like a fiddle, and the cover bolts to the frame tightly. There should be no steam escaping around the seals once it is pressurized. Turn off the heat source, allow the cooker to cool down completely, and properly reseat the top if there is one. Running a Vaseline dot around the edge of cookers in metal-on-metal design will ensure a tight fit and help shield the cover from seizure to base during use. Before each usage make sure you add a suitable measure of water to the bottom of the cooker, in any case, adequate to bring the depth to 1/2 inch. Never position items directly at the bottom of the pressure cooker, or allow them to touch the outer dividers, where temperatures are highest.

Most pressure cookers are supported by a rack or trivet intended to hold the contents over the water surface and the larger All-American models have basket-shaped liners to prevent products from direct contact with the cooker itself. Let the pressure cooker slowly begin to come up to temperature. Excessively quick or lopsided heating can cause containers to burst or crack. Until closing the stopcock, always bring the cooker to a full head of steam to displace cooler air pockets. That may take a moment, particularly on larger cookers. Before shutting the door, you should see a strong flux of steam coming from the stopcock tube. Never leave unattended an under-pressure cooker. The pressure and temperature inside a cooker can change unpredictably, particularly during the initial heating periods, before the cooker still doesn't seem to be leveling fully. It is important that the cooker remain at the ideal pressure for the full cycle in order to prevent a blast and guarantee complete sanitization. Check it at regular intervals or so to ensure it is not under-or overheating and vary the source of heat. Just allow the cooker to cool slowly and all by itself. Never touch the outside of the cooker when pressurized, and do not use cold water to cool it even faster. This can cause the cooker to implode and its contents to discharge savagely. It will generate a large measure of risky energy, at any rate. Wrap an alcohol-splashed paper towel around the valve before venting it to release any residual pressure to prevent unsterile air from being drawn into the pressure cooker upon opening. Pressure cookers are potentially dangerous things. They produce high temperatures and vapor that can cause injury. Like a very sharp blade, a pressure cooker is an apparatus that demands consideration and alertness and consequently gives a great advantage.

Petri Dishes

Petri dishes are shallow, transparent plastic or glass dishes with a baggy spread. They arrive in a variety of sizes, yet the most useful size for parasitic cultures is 100 x 15 mm. Reusable glass or Pyrex dishes are long enduring and autoclavable yet are generally costly. Pre-sterilized dispensable polystyrene dishes come in sleeves of 20 or 25. They are practical, yet since they are intended to be used just once and afterward discarded, they aren't actually earth cordial. The two types of Petri dishes can be re-sterilized utilizing hydrogen peroxide and a microwave:

1. Wash the plates altogether with dishwashing cleanser, taking unique care to totally expel any residual agar.

2. Pour a small measure of 3% peroxide into each dish and whirl it around to open it to the whole inside surface of the plate. Repeat with its spread and place it on the dish.

3. Put the pile of dishes in the microwave and heat at medium force until all the peroxide has been powered off on the plates.

4. Immediately use the plates or place them in a perfect plastic bag until appropriate.

This technique is ideally paired with the use of peroxide in cultivations of agar. Use pre-sterilized plastic or autoclaved glass dishes is safer when working with agar which lacks peroxide. We recommend the addition of hydrogen peroxide to your cultures at any point imaginable to reduce sullying and allow you to work with agar in a not exactly perfect condition.

In any case, peroxide, for example, cannot be used in specific circumstances when producing spores. In these cases, we find that plaques with a diameter of 50 mm are easier to keep clean, due to their reduced surface area. You can use 4-ounce jam jars or similar heatproof glass containers if the Petri dishes are unavailable. They have the advantage to be reusable but lack clear lids and take up more than twice as much space as plates for the community.

Media Flasks

Media flasks are used for holding fluid media during sanitization and pouring Petri plates. Any thick-walled, autoclavable glass jug will do, however, attempt to find one with a generally restricted neck to encourage pouring. One and a half-liter squeezed apple or shimmering water bottles with screw top caps are ideal for this reason.

Mason Jars

We use standard Ball-style mason canning jars, generally in quart sizes. They are readily accessible, strong, and can be reused uncertainly. For grain spawn, limited mouth (70 mm) quart jars are ideal. In the event that you need to attempt the so-called "PF" method, you'll need straight-sided, half-16 ounces jam jars.

A note of alert: mason jars are solid; however, they do sometimes break. Always review them intently before use for cracks, dispose of suspicious-looking ones immediately, and be extra careful when shaking jars of grain. Don't smack them down onto the palm of your hand to separate the grains; a cracked jar can take a finger directly off. Instead, simply hold the jar by the lid end and shake it here and there. In the event that the grain is really firmly bound, and you should break it up persuasively, carefully hit the jar against a spotless towel supported by a thick cushion or against a halfway used move of pipe tape until it slackens up. (Make sure that the lid is firmly fixed too; you don't need your precious spawn flying all over the place.) Always permit your pressure cooker to heat up steadily; fast heating can cause jars to crack because of the temperature distinction between their insides and outsides.

Mason Jar Lids

Don't mess with the metal lids given in two pieces; spare those for canned tomatoes. We use a one-piece plastic lid for culture work, which is heat-resistant and modified easily to allow the legal exchange of gas. The ball makes a "Stockpiling Cap" plastic. Even though the bundling notes that these caps are "not for storage," they are simply autoclavable. You will carefully bore or cut an I-inch gap in the focal point of each cap to alter those lids. When fitted with a filter circle (see next section), these modified caps enable gasses (not yet contaminants) to go through the jar all over, so that your cultures can breathe freely.

Filter Disks

Placed between the lid and the jar's mouth, filter plates allow the exchange of gases without contaminants being exposed. They are made of a heat resistant synthetic fiber and can be regularly sterilized. They are a couple of millimeters thick and come pre-cut to match the correct jar-and-lid mix. Occasionally, when in contact with soil or form spores, they discolor. In that case, simply drill them on a medium-term basis in a 1/4-quality fade arrangement (i.e., 1/4-CUP standard quality dye in 3/4-Cup water) unlike these plates, an affordable option is Tyvek, which can be cut to fit over the jar lid. Tyvek is a synthetic material that is used in a range of applications.

Building supply stores will purchase rolls, and smaller quantities are available to Ups or the U.S. for nothing. Mail station like those oversized, indestructible envelopes for mailing. Beca using Tyvek is thinner and more flexible than the business filter plates, it should be cut more deeply around and around than the jarhead, and one inch will hang off the edge of the jar. Tyvek is also reusable but should be discarded after three or four applications.

Spawn Bags

Otherwise known as filter repair bags, these are transparent, heat-resistant, gusseted flexible plastic bags used to hold large spawning amounts. They are autoclavable and have on one side a small square filter for exchanging air. They are stacked with soil, sterilized, immunized, and fixed with an impulse (heat) sealer afterward. They are suitable for growing out large quantities of spawn because they are versatile, and it is possible to control or analyze the interior contents for pollutants without effort. They lose their heating versatility and are generally good for solitary use only, but bags fit as a fiddle can be completely cleaned out and sterilized again.

We've seen farmers use "oven bags" (or spawns) in the grocery store. While these are autoclavable and can be made to work, they lack a filter repair that doesn't exactly provide an ideal exchange of gas, and they're too small to even think about seal heating. One way to equip this sort of bag with some breathability is to wrap its neck tightly around a thick wad of polyfill or cotton and seal it firmly with a significant breathability

Impulse Sealer

Impulse sealers are used for fixing spawn bags. Make certain to get one wide enough to straddle the whole bag when extended flat, at any rate, 12 inches across. E-Bay is a good place to search for bargains on impulse sealers.

Alcohol Lamp

This is a glass lamp with a cotton wick and metal neckline. Loaded up with scouring alcohol, it gives a spotless fire to disinfecting surgical tools and inoculation loops as you work.

Then again, you can use a:

Mini torch

Sold in kitchen supply houses for caramelizing the outside layer on creme Brule, and sold in gadgets stores for soldering, these smaller than usual butane lights are useful for disinfecting tools as you work. A good quality one will have a solid base to keep it upstanding while it sits on the seat top.

Balance

Mechanical or electronic models are similarly good. The important characteristics to search for in a balance are precision to in any event 0.5 g, the ability to weigh up to at least 250 g (1 kg is better) and a dish sufficiently large to suit oversized items.

Surgical blade

Surgical blades are used for cutting and moving agar and tissue cultures. A thin-handled dismembering surgical tool with dispensable #10-sized sharp edges is ideal. If you can't find these, an all-aluminum Xacto-style blade will work OK, however, it tends to be to some degree harder to move into tight spaces.

Inoculation Loop

This wire loop toward the end of a metal or wooden handle is used to move spores or small measures of mycelium to agar plates. It very well may be found in logical or brew making supply stores or made from a dowel and a bit of thin solid wire.

An inoculation loop isn't required in the event that you use the "cardboard circle" method of spore germination.

Sharpies

This perpetual compose anyplace markers are essential for naming culture containers of all kind.

Pipes

It is useful to have two types of plastic or metal channels: a thin necked one for pouring fluids and fine powders, and a wide-mouthed one for filling jars.

Estimating [Serological) Pipette and Rubber Bulb

If you intend to work with agar, you'll need some way of estimating small volumes of fluid (1-15 mL) to add to your cultures. Ten-milliliter glass estimating pipettes are ideal for this purpose since they are autoclavable, reusable, and have markings on them to effortlessly determine volume. An elastic bulb is used to draw and administer fluids from the pipette. Both can be found at logical providers and some home mix stores. A glass 10-milliliter graduated chamber or a set of metal estimating spoons can be used for this purpose, however, it will require even more handling and care to avoid polluting your cultures while you work.

Graduated Cylinders

These are used to accurately quantify fluids. Cylinders in l-liter, 1 00-milliliter, and 10-milliliter sizes should consider every contingency.

Measuring cups and spoons

Measuring cups and spoons can be used in place of graduated tubes but are less precise to some degree. For l-cup (250rnl) to 8-cup (2 L) numbers, use Pyrex ones, and for smaller amounts use metal ones. Where sterility is needed before use, the two types can be autoclaved or sterilized in boiling water (5 minutes at a moving boil).

Syringes

Syringes are used to do mass inoculation in spore, a system called "Psilocybe Fanaticus." Ten-or twenty-milliliter sizes are used, including large bore needles (18-measure). In a pressure cooker, they may be autoclaved twice, or sterilized in boiling water. From cautious and veterinary retail shops, and from some online vendors of mushroom supplies, syringes can be purchased.

In any event, their contract is regulated in various U.S. states, and they can be elusive locally at times. When you buy spore syringes pre-filled, after use, clean and spare the syringe and needle. They are autoclavable and normally reusable.

Supplies

Hydrogen Peroxide (3%)

This antiseptic is added to cultures to shield them from defilement. It is accessible at most pharmacies or grocery stores. The real convergence of hydrogen peroxide arrangements sometimes fluctuates, so make sure the date on the bottle is of late vintage (See sidebar underneath for a method of finding hydrogen peroxide's focus level). Right now, is generally harmless to human health and requires no unique handling methods, besides wearing gloves. It is a mellow fading operator, so be careful not to dribble it onto clothing.

Increasingly concentrated (8-35%) arrangements are accessible from a variety of sources, for example, pool supply stores, and on the web. Hydrogen peroxide in focuses greater than 3% can cause severe consumes and is potentially combustible, so be careful when working with it. Peroxide corrupts reasonably quickly, to protect that it stays at the correct focus, use the bottle at the earliest opportunity subsequent to opening. Between uses, envelop the neck and cap by parafilm or plastic wrap, and store the bottle inside a spotless plastic bag in the cooler. Prior to each use, wipe down the outside of the bottle and cap (counting the mouth and neck beneath the cap) with alcohol, and take uncommon care not to touch any piece of the bottle itself with your hands or tools while apportioning. Always sanitize pipettes and graduated cylinders that will come into contact with peroxide before use, either in a pressure cooker along with your media or by submerging them in boiling water for 5 minutes.

Isopropyl [Rubbing] Alcohol

This is used for sanitizing hands, surfaces and containers, and as fuel for alcohol lamps. It is accessible in grocery stores and pharmacies in either 70% or 91 % focuses, both of which is reasonable. Cautioning: Isopropanol is profoundly combustible!! Get it far from open blazes, if you don't mind make sure whatever alcohol you have used has completely evaporated before you light your alcohol lamp.

Blanch

Standard quality laundry dye is useful for cleaning surfaces and tools. Avoid brands with added cleansers. Weaken to in any event 1/4 quality before use. A 10% quality arrangement in a spray bottle is an excellent surface and air disinfectant.

Parafilm

Parafilm is a paraffin-based, flexible film utilized to seal Petri dishes. It is gas permeable, which means that it takes into account gas exchange while keeping contaminants out of cultures. An advantageous form in 1-inchwide rolls is sold by some garden supply vendors as "Uniting Tape." If you can't find Parafilm, you can substitute polyethylene stick film, for example, Glad Wrap (yet not Saran Wrap or similar brands, which are made from polyvinylchloride and are not gas permeable.). Utilizing a sharp blade, carefully cut a 1-to 2-inch-wide segment off the end of a full roll.

Surgical Gloves

Dispensable latex gloves are essential for getting grimy hands far from your perfect cultures. They need not be pre-sterilized. Simply wash your hands and arms a long time before putting them on, at that point wipe the outside of the gloves with an alcohol-drenched paper towel (always permit them to dry totally before going anyplace close to an open fire.)

Substrates & Casing Materials

Whole Grains

For spawn creation, the most commonly used substrate is entire grain. Entire grains make an ideal mechanism for spawn for a number of reasons. Each grain demonstrations like a smaller than normal capsule of supplements, minerals, and water that is handily colonized by higher fungi, while its sinewy husk halfway shields it from contamination by different living beings. Upon colonization, the grains are effectively separated from each other. At long last, when colonized grain spawn is used to immunize mass substrates, each grain fills in as a minimal container of mycelium and supplement holds, a remote station from which the fungus can leap off onto the new medium.

While practically any cereal grain will work as spawn, we recommend delicate winter (white) wheat, since it has worked well for us, and is by all accounts liberated from the bacterial contaminants that can be present on rye and different grains. You may use whatever grains are readily accessible to u, however we do suggest utilizing larger bit grains like rye, wheat, or corn, instead of small-grained cereals like millet or rice, which tend to cluster together when cooked. We have seen a few growers use wild birdseed mix with good results, which has the undeniable bit of leeway of being modest and readily accessible. Be that as it may, because it is a mixture of various sized grains, birdseed is increasingly difficult to moisten appropriately. It can likewise be very clingy when damp. To limit these issues, hydrate birdseed with a 24-hour cold soak instead of boiling water, and flush and drain it very well before stacking into containers. You should attempt to use natural grains at whatever point conceivable, since that is the best way to guarantee that they have not been treated with fungicides.

Malt Extract, Dried

This is a powdered extract of grains that have been "malted" or developed to advance the incomplete transformation of their starch into sugars. Malt extract is used as an important substitute in agar products. It is readily accessible from preparing suppliers. Make sure to use light or tan malt. Darker malts have been caramelized and fungi are not growing well on caramelized sugars.

Yeast Extract

A dried extract of yeast cells, plentiful in vitamins, minerals, and protein, yeast extract is added to agar media as a wholesome enhancement. Brewer's yeast, accessible in numerous health food stores, is an adequate substitute, however it isn't as effective as evident yeast extract.

Calcium Carbonate [CaCO3]

Calcium carbonate is otherwise called lime, hydrated lime, limestone flour, clam shell flour, and chalk. It is used to cradle the pH of packaging soils and substrates, demoralize contamination, and give calcium to the growing fungus. Fungi tend to prefer slightly fundamental (for example pH > 8) media, while microbes and some different contaminants don't. Check the name to be certain the calcium carbonate you buy is low in magnesium « 1 %), because a few fungi don't grow well on substrates containing high measures of it.

Calcium Sulfate

Also called gypsum, calcium sulfate is used to capture overabundance water in substrates, making them simpler to shake or separate, and assisting with preventing water logging and contamination. It is essentially impartial in pH and has no buffering capability.

Hardwood Sawdust and Chips

These are substrates for the genus Psilocybe cyanescens, P. azurescens and related lignicolous species (wood-possessing). Birch, cottonwood, oak, birch, and beech are suitable, though most hardwood species will do so. In case you have any of these tree species growing nearby, you might have the option to get fresh chips from your nearby highway office or garden focus, or you might be able to chip your own. Chips developed in winter or late winter from trees are best as they will be highest in sugars and contain at least green matter, which can be a contamination vector in beds.

You can sometimes get local hardwood chips from grill vendors, who market them for use in food smokers. If you don't tackle hardwoods locally, you can buy wood chips online. Fine chipped wood beech or maple chips are marketed as creature bedding (Beta-Chip and SaniChip are two brands to pay special attention to), yet they are usually too fine to even suggest using alone, and need to be paired with larger chips or something to affect them.

Sawdust Fuel Pellets

Used for home heating in special wood stoves, these are made from sawdust compressed into tiny pellets. During production, the high heat generated: makes them pretty sterile. The pellets fall into sawdust once more when they are moistened with warm water. This item is available at home heating suppliers as well as some home improvement stores. Stove pellets make a good source of sawdust for substrates-just make sure to get a brand made from hardwoods only. In a number of tree species, including birch and oak, they are additionally sold as fuel to food smokers.

Spiral-Grooved Dowels

Spiral-grooved dowels are readily accessible from woodworking providers as furniture-joining pegs; the best ones for mushroom use are 1 to 2 inches long and 1/4-inch or 5/16-inch in diameter. They are normally made from birch and will be assigned thusly. They are most commonly utilized in mushroom cultivation on logs, where the colonized pegs are beat into openings around the perimeter of the log. The spiral furrow around the outside of the peg gives a maximal surface area from which the mycelium can leap off onto resulting substrates.

Paper Pellet Cat Litter

Used for the capacity of cultures in small glass tubes. The free, open structure and restricted nourishing content of paper makes it ideal for the long-term maintenance of most mushroom species. Search for a brand that is unscented and made of 100% reused paper; Crown, Good Mews, and Yesterday's News are three brands we have found to be effective.

Peat Moss

A component of casing soil, peat moss is sold in garden focuses all over the place. While it has minimal healthy benefit, its high-water holding capacity gives dampness to the creating fruitbodies. It is to some degree acidic and must be cradled with calcium carbonate.

Vermiculite

Vermiculite is another component of casing soil. It is used for its water holding capacity, and its soft, open structure, which permits appropriate gas exchange. It is accessible at many garden providers. Use the coarsest grade you can find. There is a fantasy that vermiculite contains asbestos, which isn't valid. Apparently, there was a solitary vermiculite mine in Montana that was debased with asbestos, and it was closed. After this episode was publish moss and vermiculite. Different manufacturers started testing their vermiculite for asbestos, yet it was not found anyplace else. In any case, vermiculite and similar materials (like peat and calcium salts) do contain a great deal of extremely fine particulates, which can be harmful whenever breathed in. Always wear a painter's residue veil when handling them in their dry state.

Water Crystals

Made from a synthetic polymer chemically similar to super paste, these crystals can maintain their weight in water by 400 times, and then slowly discharge it back into their atmosphere. We feel like smooth gelatin when fully hydrated. These are used to track water use in agriculture and gardening and to prevent plants from drying out completely between watering. These are added to the casing soil in mushroom cultivation to help maintain sufficient levels of humidity. The crystals come in two assortments: the ones made from potassium sodium or others. Since elevated sodium levels are harmful to multiple fungi, make sure to get the potassium-made version. (One brand based on potassium is called "Land Sorb").

Spores

Obviously, none of any of these materials are of any use to you in the event that you don't have mushroom spores to grow on them. Why at that point, you ask, didn't we disclose to you first where to get your hands on some Psilocybe spores?

It's a good inquiry, and one that requires an entangled answer, tragically. Almost certainly you live in a country that has (anyway strange the notion) regarded these unassuming and delicate mushrooms illegal. While the specialists can do little to genuinely contain these life forms (no more so than if they somehow managed to boycott the shape growing on your shower drapery), they could detain you for horsing around with them. That is a pitiful truth worth contemplating for a moment before you choose to do as such. If, at last, you conclude that the prizes exceed the risks (as we accept, they do), we ask you to practice alert while doing a/1ything unlawful. Stay under the radar; be prudent. Don't converse with others about your new hobby (or if nothing else not except if you know for total sure they are "cool"). Think of conceivable elective implications for your buys, regardless of whether you just instruct them to yourself: the 50-pound bag of w) 1eat berries is to crush your own bread flour, the malt is for your next clump of home brewed chocolate watchman, etc. Don't gloat about your endeavors on the Internet; anyway, mysterious you think you are anything you do online nowadays can be followed back to your PC, if somebody needed to. It may require a court request, however it's despite everything better not to face the challenge. Do not begin this hobby with the notion that instantly you'll turn into the neighborhood psychedelic mushroom boss, a parasitic Tony Montana. The benefit thought process has driven endless individuals adrift, as it might you be able to.

CHAPTER 4
PF TEK Improved

In this chapter, along with our refinements of it, we describe the popular "Psilocybe Fanaticus" mushroom cultivation technique, otherwise known as the "PF Tek." This method is the first system to be exposed to for many Psilocybe mushroom growers nowadays, so we felt it was important that we cover it in our book, even if we don't recognize it as a general practice. Since it is as similar to foolproof as a method of growing mushrooms can get, it is a good starting point for a beginner. It requires a minimum investment of time and expense, and in a relatively short time exposes the novice to the whole life cycle of a mushroom. Taking a close and first-hand look at this process will allow you to understand the principles that underlie the more complex procedures that follow. If you choose to start your mushroom cultivation with a Psilocybe cubensis spore-water syringe rather than a spore print, this method is a good way to use it (although not the only one: you could also use it to directly inoculate grain spawning. The technique allows you to very quickly produce a pure fruiting strain of P. cubensis, with minimal interference. Above this is placed a thin layer of dry vermiculite, followed by a few layers of aluminum foil. The brown rice flour provides the colonization of the fungus with a healthy nutrient base, while the vermiculite acts as a reservoir for water and helps create an open, airy structure that allows the growing crops to breathe. The jars are then sterilized in a pressure cooker or bath with boiling water. Upon cooling, the first layer of foil is removed, and at various points around the jar's diameter the jars are easily filled with a few milliliters of a spore solution from a syringe. The top layer of foil is replaced, and the jars are then placed in an incubator or a warm, draft-free spot. With time the spores will germinate and fuse to form a dikaryotic mycelium with an appropriate mate.

In each injection, the large number of spores ensures that mating will occur and that each jar contains a wide variety of strains. The many strains present are competing to colonize the jar, with the weaker ones being overtaken by the most vigorous (and by extension, most likely to well bear fruit). The jars should be completely colonized after some weeks or so and are ready to be fruited. The "cakes" of mycelium are knocked out of the jars at this point in the original PF Tek and placed upside down on a bed of moistened perlite at the bottom of a clear container such as an aquarium or a plastic storage bin, which is covered to maintain high humidity levels. The fruiting chamber is placed under a light source (fluorescent lights grow connected to a timer or even a brightly illuminated window). Once or twice a day, the cover is removed, and the cakes are fanned by hand to remove built-up C02, then misted with water from a hand spray bottle. In time, primordia form on the cake's outer surface and eventually ripen into full-sized mushrooms. We leave the substratum in the jar in our "improved" PF Tek, and mushrooms fruit only from the top surface of the jar. This serves a series of ends. One, it eliminates the need for perlite tubs which are elaborate and messy. Instead, the jars are perforated into any clear enclosed container, or even a plastic bag, to allow exchange of gas.

Second, the need for high ambient humidity is reduced, because the top layer of pure vermiculite acts as a casing layer, holding a reservoir of water that can be drawn from the developing fruits. Because fruiting is confined to a horizontal surface, the forming mushrooms retain a much more natural appearance and form. On the other hand, the original "cake" approach tends to produce fruits of odd shapes and sizes, as they grow around the cake at random points. (Since spores are most efficiently dispersed from downward-facing gills, most mushrooms utilize gravity to orient themselves horizontally. If, as in our method, the stipes are already pointing in the right direction, they naturally grow straight and tall.) By incorporating a casing layer, the "improved" PF Tek resembles more closely the advanced methods that we later present. You'll be more than familiar with the basic mushroom life cycle after you've performed this method once or twice, and ready to move on.

The "Improved" PF Tek

Materials 40 mL (meager '/4 cup) natural brown rice flour (per jar)

140 mL ('/2 cup) vermiculite (per jar), in addition to extra for casing layer

Water 1/2-16 ounces (250 mL) mason jars Aluminum foil Spore-water syringe(s)

Alcohol lamp or butane lighter Rubbing alcohol

Material Notes: Brown rice flour is accessible at some health food stores, or you can pound your own in a little coffee processor or zest factory. The jars ought to be straight sided Gelly jars), without the shoulders present on larger-sized canning jars. Faucet water is fine; however, you can use bottled or refined if your water source is suspect.

Sterilization Note: This method contains the one occurrence right now we depict a boiling water shower cleansing of a substrate as a choice to pressure-cooking. The water shower process is effective, yet not 1 00% reliable; some percentage of jars prepared with it will at present be likely to taint. In the event that you have a pressure cooker, you should use it here as well; if not, presently is as good a time as any to get one.

1. Depending on the number of jars you will vaccinate (a 10 mL syringe contains enough answer for immunize 8-10 jars), place the necessary measure of vermiculite in a bowl. Presently evacuate around 5% of this and place it in a separate container.

2. Into the principle bowl of vermiculite, add water a little at a time, mixing as you go, until the mixture can't hold any longer and tl1ere is only a slight overabundance of water at the bottom of the bowl. Presently add the held dry material and mix completely. The vermiculite should now be at "field capacity," implying that it contains the most extreme measure of water it can easily hold.

3. Empty the brown rice flour into the bowl and mix well, covering the vermiculite grains with a layer of moistened flour.

4. Spoon this mixture into the jars, leaving a level 1/2-inch (1-centimeter) hole at the top. Place it into the jars freely and don't pack it down; keeping an open, breezy structure will permit the mycelium to breath and grow at an ideal rate. Take a clammy paper towel and wipe down the sides and around within edges of the jars to completely expel any wanderer substrate, which could somehow turn into a source of contamination.

5. Occupy the rest of the space of the jar with dry vermiculite. This layer will at first go about as a hindrance to contaminants, which, should they by one way or another find their way inside the jar, would be prevented from coming into contact with the substrate.

Afterward, it will fill in as the casing soil, from which the mushrooms will fruit.

6. Take two 5-inch square bits of aluminum foil and wrap them firmly over the mouth of the jar. Freely screw lids onto the jars, taking care not to tear the foil beneath. (The use of lids in the PF Tek is discretionary yet provides an additional layer of assurance.)

7. Burden the jars into your pressure cooker, along with the proper measure of water, and sanitize the jars at 15 psi for 45 minutes. If there is sufficient room, the jars might be stacked in more than one layer.

Or then again (Boiling Water Bath Method):

8. Place the jars in a large cooking pot in a solitary layer, along with enough water to bring it to about halfway up the sides of the jars. Spread the pot and boil for 1 .5 hours. Check once in a while to make sure the water level stays steady, adding water as vital.

Phase 2: PF Tek Inoculation

1. When the jars have cooled down to room temperature, put them on a clean working surface, together with the spore-water syringe and alcohol lamp. Replace the lids and drop the cover over the top foil.

2. Remove the cover from the syringe, rub the needle with a moistened alcohol, clean paper towel or cotton ball, and place the tip of the needle in your lamp's flame until it begins glowing red (be careful to keep the plastic end of the needle away from the flame, and be careful when using alcohol near an open flame).

3. Using one container at a time, removing the top layer of tape, shaking the syringe gently to disperse the spore solution, and injecting a small amount into the jar at four equally spaced dots right inside the inner rim. Insert 1

inch (2 cm) of needle into the jar so its point passes the dry layer of vermiculite, then squeeze out a few drops. You should be in a spot to see the solution run down the jar sides. Repeat on three points left. Every jar should get 1-1, 5 mL total solution.

4. Inject all the jars in the same way, covering the top layer of foil and cap (if used) at each. Label the outside of the jars with relevant information and/or notebook number, and position in a clean, warm spot to incubate.

Phase 3: Incubation

The jars should be incubated in the 75-850 F range, at a warm, draft-free location. If your home temperature is consistently within this range, then it should be sufficient to simply store them in a clean box. If not, an incubator box will ensure healthy and rapid growth, and is easy to build from a cooler and a few items that you can buy from a pet store's reptile department.

Materials

- ✓ 25-50 gallon plastic or Styrofoam cooler
- ✓ 8-watt reptile heating mat
- ✓ Flexible indoor regulator controller
- ✓ Air temperature thermometer

Place the heating mat and thermometer in the cooler, plug the mat in and switch on the temperature controller. Set the controller to its lowest setting and let the cooler warm up for a few hours before switching it up step by step until it reaches a steady 80 ° or something like this. Arrange the heating mat on one side of the cooler, and stack your jars on the contrary side, as a long way from direct heat as could be allowed. Depending on the surrounding temperature of the room, you may need to incidentally alter the indoor regulator to keep a consistent temperature inside the cooler. At the point when surrounding temperatures go above 85°, you'll have to make sense of a way to shield the jars from overheating. Right now, then developing an elaborate refrigeration gadget, your most logical option is to store them in a shut container in a cool spot in your home, for example, an unheated basement. If no such place is accessible to you, this would be a good time to take a break for some time, until outside temperatures have cooled adequately to continue cultivation.

Phase 4: Germination/Colonization

Within a week or so, the first signs of spore germination in your jars will start to appear. Look for tiny pinpoints of bright white fozzy growth, usually directly below the injection points near the base of the jar. Those tiny colonies radiate outward in time to form individual mycelium spheres. The spheres inside each jar will join each other within 10 days to a few weeks, and the jar will be fully colonized.

Contamination

The jar is likely to be contaminated if you see any growth in your jars that is not pure white in color and should be removed from the incubator immediately and disposed of. Molds which tend to have highly colored spores in shades of blue, green, black or pink will be the most common offenders. On the other hand, bacterial contamination will appear as spots of wet, sticky blobs on the jar's inner surface, and may be accompanied by a sour or rotten smell of apples. Remember to always remove contaminated culture containers from your work and growing areas, and thoroughly clean the containers before returning them to your workspace.

Phase 5: Fruiting

Once the jars have colonized completely, they're ready to be fruited. At this stage, the lids and foil are removed, the top layer of vermiculite is moistened, and the jars are put under a light source, either by artificial light given by a dedicated fluorescent "grow" light or by a brightly lit window. Since P cubensis requires light to stimulate fruiting, and you want to limit fruiting to the upper surface of the cakes, you need to restrict light exposure to just that area of the jars in some way. This can be done in numerous numbers of ways, such as wrapping the jars in aluminum foil, or thick, opaque paper strips. One simple method that we used is to place the jars inside short pieces of cardboard tubing, such as the type used to store posters, cut to come just above the rim.

Preparing the Jars for Fruiting

1. Remove the lids and foil from each jar. You may see a few "fans" of mycelium jabbing up through the vermiculite layer.

2. Wipe a spotless fork with some alcohol, permit it to evaporate, and afterward delicately scratch (not scratch off) the dry vermiculite layer right down to the top of the cake underneath, to break up and equitably circulate the mycelial parts within.

3. Take a spray mister of clean water and mist the vermiculite until it is saturated (it will darken slightly in color; when you can see free streaming water, that is enough.)

4. Repeat with each jar, cleaning the fork each time to prevent inadvertently spreading contaminants.

5. At the point when the entirety of the jars is ready, place them in singular cardboard cylinders inside an encased container, for example, a large clear plastic bag (cut or perforate it to give a few gas exchange) or a reasonable plastic stockpiling tub.

6. If you are utilizing a fluorescent grow light, set your timer to an 8-hour on 1 16-hour off cycle; in any case, simply find the jars in a sufficiently bright area, for example, close to a radiant window. The ideal

temperature of your growing area ought to be in the 65-75°F range, slightly lower than that required during colonization.

7. Mist the casing lightly a few times every day to replace any water lost to vanishing.

You should see primordia begin to form within a couple of days to about fourteen days. They will no doubt grow inside the casing layer and will not be visible until small-scale mushrooms are already established all around. They tend to grow astonishingly quickly when they have accomplished this scale and may seem to arrive at full size virtually medium term. They will draw water from the cake and the casing layer as they expand, so make sure to increase misting varying to keep the vermiculite saturated, always taking care not to overwater.

Phase 6: Harvesting when the mushroom has reached a suitable size for successful spore dispersal, it stops growing and increases its cap to expose the atmosphere to its spore-providing gills. This argument is only followed by the best time to pick your mushrooms, as a single mushroom can release a galactic amount of spores, which can make things incredibly chaotic. When the mushroom prepares to reveal its gills the best way to tell is to pay close consideration to the partial veil, the thin protective film that covers them. At first, when the cap is completely inserted (looking a lot like those good old streetlamps globe-on - a-shaft), the partial veil is covered up). As the cap starts to grow, the veil forms around the cap's bottom hemisphere as a round, light-colored band.

When the cap begins to flatten out, the partial veil gets extended past its ability to expand and begins to tear, pulling away from the external edges of the gills. Eventually, the partial veil withdraws from the cap altogether, and its remainders stay joined to the stipe in a skirt-like ring, known as an annulus). Ideally, you need to pick your mushrooms when the partial veil is visible, or at the most recent, before it begins to break.

Harvesting the mushrooms is as basic as getting a handle on them at the base and winding tenderly while pulling them far up into the clouds from the casing. In the event that your fingers are small and deft enough, you can use your spotless hands to do as such; if not, a pair of clean chopsticks makes a good harvesting apparatus. Any piece of the mushroom that remaining parts behind in the casing will rot, so take care to remove everything, down to the base of the stipe. Do whatever it takes not to touch the casing layer and take uncommon care not to harm close by less-created mushrooms or primordia. Sometimes, be that as it may, it is difficult to avoid upsetting or evacuating close by mushrooms while expelling another. Right now, is smarter to remove these "babies" also, as opposed to leaving them behind. Often, upsetting them cuts off their association with the substrate and they stop growing and eventually rot. What vitality the culture would somehow, or another have expended on these fruits will be occupied to other people, so don't stress a lot over the infrequent loss.

Normally, a decent measure of vermiculite will be adhered to the base of the harvested mushrooms, leaving behind a divot in the casing layer. When you are done harvesting, simply fill these holes with fresh vermiculite, mist the casing altogether and return the jars to their fruiting area. During the period immediately following a harvest, increment misting recurrence altogether, so as to replace the substantial measure of dampness removed from the cakes.

Each jar should produce three to five yields, or flushes, of mushrooms, with about seven days of recovery time between each harvest. During the later flushes, when the supplements of the substrate are substantially drained, the cakes will shrink and pull away from the sides of the jar, uncovering the dividers of the cakes to the atmosphere and to light. Mushrooms will at that point begin to form around the sides of the cakes. Aside fro111. Being increasingly difficult to remove totally from the jar, these are not an issue (this is the place a pair of chopsticks proves to be useful).

After the fourth or fifth flush, the jars will be almost completely drained, and the number of mushrooms that form will be insignificant. Now, the cakes ought to be discarded, since the mycelium in them will begin to pass on and will eventually rot, turning into a vector for contamination.

CHAPTER 5
Working with agar

Preparing Agar Plates

Mushroom crops are usually grown out on nitrified agar plates and maintained. The agar's smooth, semi-solid surface provides an outspread, two-dimensional growth pattern, taking into account the easy evaluation of a crop and the distinctive proof of and separation from any pollutants that should arise. Agar is a polysaccharide (a sugar-like atom) found in the cell dividers of certain green growth. At the point when disintegrated in boiling water and afterward cooled, agar partially solidifies, much like gelatin.

Agar itself gives no sustenance to the fungus, so a variety of supplements are added to the medium, for example, malt sugar and yeast extract. The fixings are combined with water in a heatproof container, sterilized in a pressure cooker, and filled Petri dishes while still fluid. One of the media most commonly used is Malt-Yeast Extract Agar, or MYA, for short. It is a generally useful medium, one on which all species of Psilocybe will grow gracefully.

Senescence

Growers often interchange media recipes to avoid strain senescence, the corruption of a culture because of maturing.

Sometimes after a number of transfers between plates, a culture can begin to grow feebly, or even stop growing inside and out. Senescent cultures tend to fruit inadequately or not in the slightest degree and are typically discarded for re-separation of a healthy strain from spores.

The causes of strain senescence are yet not surely knowing; however, it appears to occur frequently when a culture is maintained on similar media recipe for a long timeframe. Fungi (like humans) appear to do best when given a variety of foods to expend, and like us they grow exhausted and even pass on when given something very similar to eat day in, day out. To avoid senescence, it is basic that you change your media recipe each time you use it, which "works out" the fungus, provoking it to produce various sets of proteins constantly. One basic way to do this is to add small quantities of grain flour to each bunch, rotating the type you use each time you pour new plates, as portrayed underneath. Once in a while, in any case, you should challenge your fungus considerably further, by requesting that it grow on a completely novel medium. This can be especially useful for restoring a culture that begins to show evidence of debilitating. Right now, need to reject every basic sugar and starches completely, and give it something completely novel to process. (We call this recipe "Anything" Agar.)

It might grow gradually on the new medium, however following half a month of growth, when you move it back to an increasingly balanced medium like MYA, it is likely to detonate with new growth. What would it be a good idea for you to feed it? Any cellulose, starch, or sugar will do, including soybeans, paper pellets, raspberry jam, nutty spread whatever you can think of. The sky's the point of confinement. We have even known about one cultivator who took care of his fungi dried crickets he found at a pet store! Now and again you may find a material that your fungi refuse to grow on. Assuming this is the case, no issue, simply take a stab at something else. Another way to avoid strain debasement is to limit the number of transfers of each culture that you perform.

- ✓ Malt Yeast Agar [MYA] Medium
- ✓ 22 g agar
- ✓ 12 g light malt extract
- ✓ 1 g yeast extract
- ✓ 1/4 tsp natural grain flour (rotate among oats, cornmeal, amaranth, rice, millet, rye or some other starch or sugar you can think of)
- ✓ 5 g wood fuel pellets or hardwood sawdust
- ✓ 1 L faucet water 8 mL 3% hydrogen peroxide (discretionary, added after sanitization and cooling; see underneath.)

1. Add every single dry fixing to jar, followed by the water. Make certain to use a jar that is 1.5 to 2 times the volume of media wanted, so it doesn't boil over during cleansing. Attachment the neck of the bottle with cotton fleece, at that point wrap the opening and neck of the bottle with aluminum foil.

2. Put the jar in the pressure cooker along with the necessary measure of water. If you will add peroxide to the agar, make certain to sterilize a few estimating pipettes too, wrapped in aluminum toil to keep up sterility before use.

3. Sterilize at 15 psi for 30 min. Try not to cook your agar media for longer than 45 minutes, since this can cause the media to caramelize, and fungi don't grow well on caramelized sugars.

4. Permit the pressure cooker to come to atmospheric pressure, at that point carefully move the jar and pipettes to a glove enclose or front of a stream hood while still hot. It is helpful to use a few layers of clean paper towel as a potholder while moving items from the pressure cooker to the workspace.

5. When using peroxide: apply 8 mL of 3 percent hydrogen peroxide, using a sterile channel e or calculating spoon, until the outside of the container is co ('} l enough to handle quickly yet very warm at the same time (between 1' 0 °-140 ° F). In the two headings, rotate the medium gently a few times to blend it in altogether. Be careful not to over-agitate it and build bubbles that end up in your dishes.

6. Open your Petri dishes sleeves as planned on the bundling and stack them directly onto your work area. To later power carry plastic jacket.

7. Operating with stacks of ten plates one after the other, raise the entire stack by the lid of the bottom plate in one hand, leaving the bottom half on the top of the table, and slowly dump just enough medium into the plate to completely cover it. Replace the stack, and repeat until complete, with the plate above. One liter of average will suffice for regular Petri dishes of 20-30 1 00 mm. Make an effort not to agitate when you pour in the mixture. When solid particles are at the bottom of the cup, leave them there; all usable nutrients should be in arrangement, and you need the media on your plates to be transparent enough to see through.

8. If you find that the agar starts to solidify before you finish pouring it, holding the jar in a shallow pot of hot (1 50 ° F) water when not being used is often beneficial.

9. Stack the finished plates in a single section, and freely replace the sleeve they came in to permit each plate in the stack to cool gradually and uniformly, limiting buildup on the upper plates (buildup can make the agar difficult to see, and can turn into a vector for contamination). A similar effect can be accomplished by covering each stack with a spotless coffee cup or substantial glass half-loaded up with hot water.

10. Permit plates to cool medium-term.

11. Peroxide plates can be left for a few days in a cool sans draft spot to additionally drive off any residual buildup. Lay them out in stacks of a few, inexactly secured with a couple of sheets of clean waxed paper. Plates without peroxide ought to be placed in sleeves when they have cooled.

12. Slide the plastic sleeve back over the plates and tape it shut firmly with clear pressing tape. Store them agar side up (to additionally limit buildup) in a cool and dry place until required.

Care of Petri Dishes and Cultures

When making transfers, lids ought to be removed for as brief a time as could be expected under the circumstances, and held legitimately over the plate to keep contaminants out.

Cultures ought to be stockpiled side up too. Be that as it may, it is a good plan to give new transfers a day or so to grow out onto the new plate before flipping around them, or the moved material probably won't hold fast to the fresh agar surface. Culture plates ought to be wrapped around their edges with a few layers of parafilm.

Spore Streaking

Even if you use PF Tek to grow P. cubensis mushrooms or collect fresh specimens from the wild, you will need to start your crops from spores to isolate a strain of pure fruiting. There are two methods you can use to start cultivation of mushrooms from spores to agar. A sterile inoculating loop is used in the conventional system to extract a small measure of the spores from a print, and then streaked over an agar plate. Remember that you cannot use Petri plates containing peroxide for this reason, as it would slaughter the spores. On the other side, spores are sprouted in clean cardboard circles in an innovative process developed by Rush Wayne and illustrated in volume two of his book Growing Mushrooms the Easy Way.

This method gives a few unmistakable advantages over the traditional method. The small size of the circles and the tight openings of the test tubes help keep contaminants out of cultures that are unprotected by peroxide. In addition, it is a genuinely fast system: the circles are immediately colonized and would then be able to be placed legitimately onto peroxidated agar.

Finally, because the circle demonstrations both as the substrate and as the instrument used to lift spores from the spore print, it accommodates a proficient exchange, which is particularly helpful when the spore print is black out and light on spores. Utilizing a punching tool, small circles are cut from thin, flat cardboard (the gray sheets found at the back of stack of paper are great). These are moistened slightly, placed in a jar and sterilized along with test tubes containing 5-10 drops of a malt-yeast extract solution. At the point when cool, the circles are used to pick up a small amount of spores, and afterward dropped into the tube, where they ingest the malt solution. In time, the spores develop and when the modest circles are fully colonized, they are transferred to peroxide agar plates.

Agar Spore Germination

This method is indistinguishable from the one used when making spore-water syringes, apart from that here the spores are transferred to sans peroxide agar plates instead of water.

Materials

- ✓ Spore print
- ✓ Sans peroxide agar
- ✓ Petri dishes
- ✓ Inoculating loop
- ✓ Alcohol lamp

Parafilm

1. Heat the inoculation loop inside the alcohol lamp in your glove box or flow hood until it sparks out super-hot.
2. Using your other hand to lift the lid of the first Petri dish, touch the tip of the loop to the focal point of the agar to cool it (this also places a thin agar film on the loop, which will allow the spores to stick to it).
3. Cover the plate and afterward use the loop to pick up a small number of spores from your print.
4. Streak these across the Petri dish in a S-shaped movement and afterward close the plate.
5. Re-sterilize and cool the loop before marking each plate.
6. Wrap the edges of every plate with parafilm after inoculation, mark them with any applicable information, and hatch agar side up.

Cardboard Disk Spore Germination

Materials

- ✓ Spore print
- ✓ Cardboard circles
- ✓ J/2-pint jar and lid Screw-capped test tubes or vials (2 or 3 for each spore print)
- ✓ Malt-yeast agar solution (1 tsp malt and a little pinch of yeast extract in 1 00 mL water)
- ✓ Pipette or eyedropper
- ✓ Tweezers
- ✓ Alcohol lamp

Parafilm

1. Place cardboard circles in J/2-pint jar, along with 1 - 2m1 water, and seal. Place 5-10 drops of malt solution

into test tubes and lightly seal. Sterilize the jar and tubes for 15 minutes at 45 psi and permit to cool completely.

2. Place your glove box or flow hood with all the tools and materials.

3. Heat the alcohol lamp tweezers up to high and allow to cool.

4. Open the jar and extract one circle using tweezers. Spread jar.

5. Lightly touch the edge of the circle to part of the spore print. You ought to have the option to see the black spores holding fast to the plate.

6. Open a test tube and drop the plate onto the bottom of the tube.

7. Repeat 3-5 times for every tube.

8. Create in any event two tubes of plates for every spore print.

9. Seal the tubes with parafilm and hatch.

10. At the point when the spores have sprouted and the circles are fully colonized, move a couple to singular peroxide-containing agar plates.

Incubation

Vaccinated culture plates and spore circles ought to be hatched in a warm, sans draft area, in the 75-85° F range. In the event that the temperature in your home is consistently within this range, at that point it is adequate to simply store them in a perfect box.

Tissue Transfers (Cloning)

Clean, fresh, mushrooms, either fruited from a multispore culture (from a PF Tek jar, for instance), or gathered from the wild, can likewise be used to start an agar culture. Right now, coming about culture ought to be a solitary strain and should display indistinguishable attributes from its parent. Since it is hereditarily indistinguishable from the strain from which it was secluded, it is viewed as a clone, and this procedure is known as cloning. Because of this, we generally search for the healthiest specimens in a populace to clone, with the hope of isolating a strain that will furnish consistent and dynamic fruitings with each use. Good characters to search for in a parent incorporate early, large, or thick fruits, and any that have a healthy look in general. Isolating a solitary, fruiting strain is as basic as picking the choicest specimens from your yields and culturing them on agar.

The mushrooms are torn or cut open in a glove box or flow hood, and a small piece of clean mycelium is removed from the inside of the stipe or the area of the cap simply over the gills and placed on a fresh agar plate. After a short brooding period, the mycelial fragments grow out onto the plate and would then be able to be subcultured. Often nonetheless, for unknown reasons, clones taken from a similar parent mushroom do display varying mycelial qualities.

Consequently, we make various (at least four) cultures from everyone, and spare simply the best coming about cultures for additional use. Looks can be beguiling and strains may not perform as predicted by their appearance, so we clone the same number of various specimens as time and space permits, so as to enhance our chances of achievement over the long haul. Because they have never been exposed to the outer condition, the cells on the inside of a mushroom ought to be clean (i.e., uncontaminated). To ensure sterility, be that as it may, you ought to always attempt to clone mushrooms at the earliest opportunity in the wake of picking them. If you can't use them immediately, you can store them in the ice chest in a clean Tupperware container fixed with a fresh paper towel for a couple of days, yet very little longer. Unlike while streaking spores, peroxide in the agar media will really enhance your chances of effective cloning, since it gives an additional layer of protection from contaminants. Accordingly, we strongly recommend utilizing peroxidated agar at whatever point doing tissue cultures, except if you find that the species or strain being referred to doesn't tolerate it.

Tissue Transfers

Materials Mushroom(s)

- ✓ Petri dishes (with peroxide)
- ✓ Scalpel
- ✓ Alcohol
- ✓ Alcohol lamp
- ✓ Cotton balls or paper towel

1. Before use, mushrooms for cloning should be cleaned entirely of any free casing material. If possible 2 this job should be finished away from the workplace. Preferably dealing with an alcohol-soaked cotton ball in your glove box or flow hood cleans the mushroom's outer surfaces.

2. Sterilize the alcohol lamp with scalpel. Press the mushroom delicately between your thumb and index finger, holding it at the base of the stipe. You should have the option to divide it along the centerline, and then strip the mushroom's two halves divided the long way, if possible, entirely through the cap. If it is a small example, or is not parting effectively, you can use the scalpel instead to open it. Try to avoid allowing the blade to legally touch the region from which you need to clone, as it may pose pollutants in your culture on the outer surfaces of the mushroom.

3. After each use, sterilize the cutting edge again.

4. Cut a small piece of mycelium from a reasonable area of the stipe or cap (generally at the thickest, most thickly

packed area) with your Petri dishes ready. It should be as big a chunk as might be expected under the circumstances, preferably from 3-8 mm wide and long. Be particularly careful not to cut right through to the mushroom's unsterile outer layers.

5. Lance the mycelium fragment gently onto your scalpel end. Lift the Petri dish lid in your other hand, place the fragment in the center of the agar and close the plate afterwards. (Sometimes the stringy idea of the mycelium will cause it to stick to the tip of the sharp edge of the scalpel; assuming this is the case, take a slice to cut through the fragment and push it down into the agar as you are doing as such.)

6. Repeat with at least three plates for each mushroom.

7. Seal the plates with parafilm, mark them properly, and place them in your hatchery. Store them straight up until they begin to grow out, and afterward turn around them not surprisingly. You should begin to see growth within a couple of days to seven days. From the start, the fragment will turn out to be uniformly fluffy, as its cells begin to isolate once more; eventually the mycelium will fan out from where it contacts the agar to colonize the whole plate.

Agar-to-Agar Transfers (Sub culturing)

A small piece of healthy-looking mycelium from the edge of a crop is cut out with a sterile scalpel and placed on the center of another plate to make agar-to-agar transfers. Growing cultures should be used or subcultured before the mycelium gets too close to the edge of the plate, since the outer edges of the plate will harbor pollutants, which would be protected under the progressive mycelial front, only to grow when they are moved to another media.

Any part of the propelling edge could be subcultured in the event the society is a mere strain. If it's a multi-strain culture (for example, that emerging from multispore inoculation), then you'll need to select mycelium with the ideal attributes at that point. The presence of at least two forms of mycelia within a solitary community is called sectoring. The visual appearance of a stable strain varies equally from species to species, but thick rhizomorphic development for all Psilocybe species is a good sign of general health. Consider divisions with moderate growth or wispy-looking mycelium which are less likely to produce a strain of fruiting.

Also put the agar wedge face down on the fresh plate, while making a move. That serves two major capacities. Above all, it brings the mycelium in direct contact with the agar, advancing the new plate's rapid colonization. Furthermore, by sandwiching the mycelium between two layers of agar containing peroxide, any contaminant spores or microorganisms that store away on the mycelial surface are destroyed.

Agar-to-Agar Transfers

Materials

- ✓ Agar culture (s)
- ✓ Sterile agar plates
- ✓ Scalpel Alcohol lamp

Parafilm

1. In a glove box or flow hood, remove any parafilm from the outside of your healthy culture dish.

2. Heat the edge of the scalpel in your alcohol lamp until it gleams, at that point cool it in a fresh Petri dish.

3. Holding the lid of the first culture dish slightly, cut squares or wedges of agar and mycelium from the ideal

segments of the plate, from 1/2 to 1 centimeter wide. For the good of simplicity, you may cut more than each wedge in turn.

4. To make the transfer, you have to remove the lid of the first culture plate completely. With the blade in one hand, lift the lid of the perfect plate slightly to the other side, skewer one wedge of agar from the culture plate on the tip of the blade and place it on the center of the new plate, mycelium side down.

5. Repeat on all plates, seal and imprint suitably, and place in the hatchery, upside down not surprisingly. (Wedges of agar stick well to fresh agar, permitting the plates to be altered immediately.)

Contamination

Contamination in cultivation of mushrooms is inescapable. One of the benefits of operating with the two-dimensional agar plate surface is that pollutants are readily detected and isolated from balanced cultures. Plates which offer some indication of contamination should be removed from the growing area and immediately discarded.

Every so often, it might be important to attempt to "salvage" a debased culture (in the event that you always do multiple indistinguishable transfers and keep clean work propensities, such events ought to be incredibly uncommon.) In this case, you ought to always move the culture away from its contaminants to another plate. In the event that you attempt to remove contaminants from an agar dish by cutting the intruders from the plate, you will likely just spread the contamination further. Because form spores are so handily upset, it is exceedingly difficult to avoid moving contaminants along with your culture to new plates and may take a few transfers before they are fully disposed of.

Diagnosing the Sources of Contamination on Agar

You can often determine the source of contaminants on agar by observing the example of the contamination on the plate.

1. If contamination shows up before the plates are used, it very well may be a sign of lacking disinfection of the agar, poor sterile strategy during pouring or capacity of the plates, or an inadequate convergence of peroxide in the medium.

2. If signs of contamination occur on the outrageous edges of the plate, either in singular settlements or in a total ring, it can show that non-sterile air had been drawn into the plates as they cooled. To prevent this, let the agar cool adequately before pouring it, and spread the plates with their plastic sleeve immediately in the wake of filling them.

3. Contamination beginning at the inoculation point means that either a debased parent culture or deficient cleansing of the blade or inoculation loop. Look at cultures to be transferred carefully before utilizing them and avoid utilizing any that are suspect. Always heat inoculating tools until they spark scorching.

4. Bacterial contamination shows up as disgusting, gleaming, translucent roundabout provinces, often white, pink, or yellow in color. Microbes thrive in wet situations and are effortlessly spread onto plates with overabundance buildup on their lids. Always hold up until agar has cooled adequately before pouring, let plates cool gradually in their plastic sleeve, and store them agar side up.

Long-Term Strain Storage

When you have disengaged a healthy fruiting strain, you will need some way to spread this equivalent strain for a long time, with the goal that you don't need to continually repeat the detachment procedure. Cloning from plate to plate again and again will eventually cause the strain to senesce, regardless of whether you modify your agar recipe consistently, as we recommend. Along these lines, you always need to use cultures that have been exposed to as barely any transfers as could be expected under the circumstances. To do this, you ought to create an "ace" culture of any strain you think about deserving of proliferation, as soon you distinguish it. The ace culture is then placed into refrigerated, long-term stockpiling, and subcultured varying. Cultures that are stored at standard fridge temperatures (38° F) enter a condition of suspended animation and can be restored by simply sub culturing them to a fresh plate. After a short recovery period, the culture will continue ordinary growth. We recommend putting away cultures on sterilized paper pellets in test tubes. Strains stored on agar can cease to exist out of the blue, maybe inferable from the high sugar content of the media. The wholesome content of paper is insignificant, yet apparently adequate to keep the culture healthy for long periods.

The limited mouths of test tubes are ideal for ' limiting buildup and contamination, and their small size takes into consideration easy capacity. However, in the event that you don't approach test tubes, you can use 1/2-pint mason jars or other similar small autoclavable containers. In the wake of transferring the culture to the tube and permitting it to grow out, the tubes are placed in an auxiliary container, (for example, a Ziploc bag) and stored in the refrigerator. Strains kept along these lines can stay practical for a long time, yet it is a good plan to recover cultures intermittently (when consistently or two) by sub culturing each to a plate, at that point coming back to fresh paper for additional capacity. The effects of peroxide on cultures stored for long periods are not notable and subsequently we keep it separate from our capacity media.

Paper Pellet Storage Medium

Materials

- ✓ Paper pellet feline litter
- ✓ Faucet water Test tubes or other reasonable containers

A channel

1. Moisten paper pellets to field capacity.
2. Burden inside pipe, absolute' 10' /2. Be vigilant to avoid any medium bits from the outside of the tubing. Seal for free.
3. Put the containers in your pressure cooker and sterilize in layers for 30 minutes at 15 psi. Jars, while test tubes should be put in a rack or a wire to hold them upright.
4. At the point when the cooker has come back to atmospheric pressure yet is still warm to the touch, open it, and carefully transfer the containers to your glove box and permit to cool.

Inoculating Storage Tubes

Paper pellet tubes are vaccinated similarly to Petri dishes. Because the cultures lack peroxide, and they are intended to be stored as long as possible, you should take additional care to avoid presenting contaminants while doing as such, following all the standard precautions. In addition, you ought to sterilize the neck of the inclination tube each time it is opened, by moving it in the fire of your alcohol lamp.

1. Fire the scalpel and the neck of the open tube.
2. Cut a small piece of agar out of a healthy culture and put it in the tube of the sawdust. Since the test tube necks are too limited to even consider allowing the blade to penetrate, it is easier to hold the tube on a level plane, place the wedge on the upper mass of the tube, seal it, and then thump it onto the sawdust delicately afterward.

3. Seal the jar, cover the cap or lid with a parafilm band and print it out properly.
4. Hatch until the paper is fully colonized, at that point place the tubes into an optional container, for example, a cooler bag or Tupperware container and refrigerate.

Recovering Cultures from Storage

To recover a culture from its stockpiling container, return the culture to room temperature for 48 hours, and transfer (under the standard clean conditions) a small chunk of mycelium-secured paper from the capacity container to a fresh, peroxidated agar Petri dish.

CHAPTER 6
Fruiting containers

When you have a completely colonized substratum, it must be put in a suitable container for casing and fruiting. The container you choose depends on the quantity of substrate to be fruited and can range from a small aluminum foil bread dish to a large receptacle for plastic transport. You will concentrate on 2-3 inches of substratum depth when fruiting smaller quantities of grain, and as much as 6 inches for larger quantities. Besides scale, while picking a fruiting container, there are sure features to consider. It should be made of a material that is sufficiently unbending to keep the substratum in place as it colonizes, and it should be completely opaque, allowing you to absorb light alone on the surface of the casing soil. Furthermore, the container's absolute depth should preferably be close to doubling the substratum depth to allow simple exchange of gas when opening the container for misting.

For example, a few growers use smaller, fully enclosed containers, plastic canisters with Snap-On spreads to create a moist environment. While this does work, it requires cutting or drilling holes in the container sides to allow exchange of gas, and it ensures that the top must be transparent at any rate to allow light to fall on the surface of the shell. Alternatively, we recommend using shallower, opaque containers which are then put inside the clammy, a fruiting chamber's sufficiently bright setting.

The fruiting chamber can be as straightforward as an unmistakable plastic bag perforated to allow exchange of gas, positioned nearly a sunlit window, or as complex as a multi-layered shelf device that holds multiple containers, fitted with synchronized blinding lights and a humidification.

The two types of fruiting containers that we often use are plastic dishwasher tubes, 1 1.5"x 13.5"x 5 "wide, which hold 4-8 quarter jars or one bag of grain, or 20"x Is" X 7 "deep plastic containers for larger quantities of substrates. The smaller dishpans are sold in equipment and kitchen supply stores, and the conveyor receptacles can mostly be bought at the café supply battle.

The Humidity Tent

The cased containers must be kept in a humid environment to prevent fast loss of dampness from the casing and substrate. Unlike numerous other cultivated mushrooms that require significant levels of relative humidity (90%-100%), we have found that Psilocybe cubensis does fine and dandy with much lower levels (down to 70%).As long as the container is placed in a nook that is adequately small, and the casing soil is kept very much watered, enough water will wick into the immediate environment to keep the mushrooms glad.. Smaller plate or tubs can simply be placed into clear plastic bags and tied shut.

Holes ought to be punched or cut in the top and sides of the bag to take into consideration gas exchange, with four or five 1/2-inch holes per square foot. (A few online mushroom providers sell pre-perforated bags precisely for this purpose.) The container ought to be removed from the bag during misting to help displace amassed carbon dioxide. The bags ought to be sufficiently large to oblige the growing mushrooms, which will extend as much as 8 inches over the top of the casing soil.

Larger single containers can be placed inside rearranged clear plastic storage tubes, with holes bored for gas exchange in their sides, or placed on a tented shelf frame. A variety of garden supply catalogs and online retailers sell "rising racks". These are three or four-layered lightweight racks enclosed inside a zippered plastic tent for moisture control. At the point when these make excellent individual mushroom growing fenced in areas when combined with a controlled lighting system. Can shelf can hold a few smaller containers or one transportation tank, with plenty of space to house the creating mushrooms in between each shelf.

Humidity Levels

Small fruiting containers ought to go into perforated plastic bags, single larger ones ought to go into large bags or clear tubs, and multiple larger ones can be placed on an encased grow rack. For whatever length of time that the size of the humidity chamber is firmly matched to the amount of substrate it contains, the dampness levels within ought to be genuinely easy to keep up with a more than once per day hand misting.

At the point when the casing soil is all around watered, it should wick enough water into the immediate environment to keep the growing mushrooms cheerful. In the event that the air in your growing area happens to be especially dry, you may need to fall back on a beneficial humidification system. Right now, least for the small-to-medium scale grower, the best scale is a cool mist (Impeller) style humidifier, which doesn't use heat to create humidity and, in this way, won't superfluously raise the temperatures of your trimming area. These are modest and readily accessible at most larger pharmacies and retail chains.

We have seen different growers develop entangled tubing systems for siphoning soggy air from a humidifier into a grow rack. This might be essential while fruiting large numbers of containers one after another, however in general the humidifier itself can simply be placed on one of the racks alongside the plate. Buildup will develop on the dividers of the enclosure, so it is a good plan to place a large plate beneath the rack to shield dampness from falling legitimately onto the floor. Unfilled and clean this plate often to avoid form development.

Lighting

Your lighting setup ought to likewise be scaled suitably to your fruiting area. Psilocybe mushrooms are unlike plants in their lighting requirements. They use light just to animate growth, not as a vitality source, and they just require short day by day times of it to fruit successfully. A good general guideline is that if the space is lit adequately to see well, it should support fruiting fine and dandy. A couple PF Jars or a solitary tub will require minimal in excess of a south-bound window or good encompassing electrical lighting. Larger grow racks will require an inherent lighting setup. We have found that 15-20-watt conservative bright light bulbs work dependably well and use almost no vitality.

However, they ought to be mounted outside the grow chamber (maybe mounted to a contiguous divider) to limit heating and reduce the risk of an electrical short out. Depending on the size and number of containers in the enclosure, it might be important to mount lamps at a few areas so as to avoid throwing shadows on the cultures. Electric lighting systems ought to likewise be put on timers, set to enlighten the space for 8 hours out of every day.

CHAPTER 7

Casing soil

Most cultivated species of mushrooms, like Psilocybe cubensis, can yield rich fruit only if the substratum is covered in a soil-like layer known as a casing layer. For example, peat moss or vermiculite, along with gypsum and calcium carbonate, are typically composed of non-nutritious materials with high water-holding capacities. The casing layer serves a number of important mushrooms producing capacities. The coating is helping to protect the substratum from losing its moisture to the atmosphere because of its high-water content. It provides a humid microenvironment within which the delicate primordia can develop, and it serves as a water-saving to draw on the parched mushrooms as they grow. Since the case layer takes up and discharges water like a wash, it also helps a grower to hold a bed comfortably at its ideal level of moisture thus reducing the risk of waterlogging the substratum and suffocating the fungus.

Furthermore, the amount of moisture on the particulate casing layer is often easier to "catch" than on exposed colonized soil, thereby enhancing the humidification process. Many recipes for the casing soil include mineral salts, such as chalk and gypsum. To some degree, peat moss is acidic, and mushroom mycelium often oozes acidic metabolites as they grow. Since a highly acidic atmosphere can damage the fungus and support the growth of microscopic organisms, the addition of chalk (calcium carbonate) to the casing soil helps to maintain a slightly necessary condition (a pH of 7.5-8.5). Gypsum (calcium sulfate) is added to help preserve a free, vaporous structure, and provide the developing fungus with mineral sustenance as calcium and sulfur. Assumed "water crystals" are arbitrary fixations that you can apply to your casing mix. Made of a synthetic polymer chemically associated with super paste, these crystals can assimilate 400 times their weight in water, and then slowly discharge it back into their atmosphere. They look like crisp gelatin when fully hydrated.

They are used to monitor water use in agriculture and gardening, and to protect plants from drying out completely between watering. Similarly, the addition to a casing layer of only a small amount of water crystals would serve to keep it hydrated and reduce the need for steady misting. A single flush of mushrooms will ransack a considerable amount of water from the casing and substratum, and these crystals can give your cultures an extra degree of protection from drying out. Despite being a synthetic substance, water crystals have been tested and shown to be non-harmful and kindhearted to the environment. We absolutely convert to carbon dioxide and water after some time. We have even been experimentally tested for protection when used in growing mushrooms. Catch mushrooms (Agaricus bisporus) grown in their presence have not been shown to corrupt or introduce the gel's chemical constituents.

The crystals come in two assortments: ones made from sodium or others made from potassium. Since significant levels of sodium are harmful to numerous fungi, make certain to get the kind made from potassium. Because the crystals debase when heated, they should be added in the wake of disinfecting or sanitizing the casing soil. While a few growers recommend sanitizing casing soils before use to limit contaminations, we have found this progression pointless as long as the components are kept perfect and dry in the first place. Nonetheless, in the event that you need to be extra careful or you find that you do experience difficulty with contamination in your casing, a brisk sanitization may help. A basic method for sanitizing small quantities uses a microwave oven. Simply place the sodden, Prepared box soil in a heat-proof container or bag (wide oven bags, the kind used to cook turkeys, or large plastic cooler bags are ideal) and microwave it on high for about 15 minutes. Make sure the bag or bottle is left unsealed to avoid blasting. Enable the bag to sit for 10 minutes, then microwave for another 15 minutes afterwards. If you do not have a microwave, you can also sterilize it at 15 psi for 45 minutes in a pressure cooker or prepare it for 2 hours in a 3500 oven. Before using allow to cool absolutely. You may need to add more water to restore the casing soil to field capacity, as it will certainly force some moisture off after heating. We've provided three simple casing recipes, just to give you a sense of the varieties used and to leverage the resources that you might have readily available.

While they are all similarly effective in cultivating P cubensis, for a number of reasons we prefer the pure vermiculite formula. It is incredibly simple, for example. Coarse vermiculite is easy to remove from the base of the harvested mushrooms, in contrast to other casing materials. Vermiculite is created by a high-heat process, so it is exceptionally clean, completely contamination-resistant and does not need to be sanitized before I use. Most significantly, because vermiculite is an inorganic substance, it does not give the fungus any sustenance. Accordingly, overlay, a condition in which the casing is over colonized by mycelium and tightly' locked together, occurs with its use infrequently. Note: The dust from inhaled vermiculite is considered to be toxic to the lungs. The residual veil of a painter should be worn for health and wellbeing when it is first opened and played with. It avoids discharging dust when the vermiculite is moistened and is never risky again.

Casing Soil Recipes

(All formulas are given on a by volume proportion.)

- ✓ Pure Vermiculite
- ✓ 10 parts coarse vermiculite
- ✓ '/2 section gypsum ($CazS04$)
- ✓ 1/2 section chalk ($CaC03$)
- ✓ Peat Moss Casing
- ✓ 10 parts peat moss
- ✓ 1/2 section gypsum ($CazS04$)
- ✓ '/2 section chalk ($CaC03$)
- ✓ "50/50" Mix
- ✓ 5 parts peat moss
- ✓ 5 parts coarse vermiculite
- ✓ 1/2 section gypsum ($Ca2S0,$)
- ✓ 1/2 section chalk ($CaC03$)

To every one of these formulas, you may add 1/2-teaspoon water crystals per liter or quart of casing soil. Always add these after any discretionary heat treatment. Regardless of which recipe you choose to use, the method of preparation is similar to that used in the PF Tek to bring the material to field capacity. Despite the fact that colonized substrates and casing soils are less dependent upon contamination than prior stages of growth, it is always a good plan to wear gloves and keep your workplace, tools, and containers as clean as could be expected under the circumstances.

1. Completely mix all the fixings together in a large, alcohol-sterilized container.

2. Save approximately 10 percent of this mixture.

3. Add water to the rest of it is saturated, and you simply begin to see free flowing water.

4. Add back the held dry mixture. In the event that appropriately moistened, pressing a handful of the soil should yield a couple of drops of water. Sterilize or sanitize whenever desired and permit to cool completely. Test an example to make sure that it remains adequately moistened and add water if necessary.

5. Add water crystals Ch tsp per liter/quart), whenever desired.

6. Apply the casing a little at once to the substratum, thereby making the layer as even as reasonably expected. To hold the framework open and breezy stop pushing it hard. The last layer should have a thickness from 1/2 inch to 1 inch.

The container should be placed immediately under fruiting conditions, inside a bag or enclosure underneath the lights after the casing layer has been applied. Mist it gently and regularly using a hand sprayer filled with a solution of 0.3% peroxide (1 section 3% H_2O_2 combined with 9 parts water), set to produce a mist as fine as might be required under the circumstances. The water requirements of the fungus are negligible during the case colonization stage and spraying on more than one occasion per day should be sufficient to offset any loss due to vanishing. Be careful not to water it too vigorously or too deeply. Watering the layer of the casing gently and often is better, as opposed to soaking it at the same time which may appear to mat it down. The mycelium will begin to infiltrate the layer of the casing before long, jabbing up through it in places where it is thinner than others. Apply additional quantities of moistened casing soil for fixing these spots with a clean knife, so that colonization of the entire layer can proceed as equally as planned under the circumstances.

Overlay forming mycelium within the layer of the casing. Small amounts of additional casing soil can fill in the denser growth areas to allow even growth across the entire sheet. It is generally best if primordia form deep within the casing layer as opposed to on top of it, to prevent overlay issues. Overlay occurs when vegetative (i.e., non-fruiting) mycelium is allowed to colonize the entire layer of the casing, which at this point turns out to be firmly bonded. Water and gases are impervious to an overlaid casing dirt, and the mycelium within it bites the dust before long.

The most ideal way to avoid overlay is to start fruiting immediately in the wake of casing, and to make sure that the ideal conditions for fruiting are present from the start. Overlay is destined to occur when the air is stuffy, humid, and the greater part of all, excessively warm. Fruitbody inception occurs when the mycelium in the casing senses a temperature and humidity contrast between the substrate and the encompassing atmosphere.

As it grows from the substrate into the casing, it eventually arrives at a boundary where moisture and temperature levels fall, implying to the mycelium that the vegetative stage is finished, and the time has come to begin fruiting. Exceptionally high humidity and warmth prevent the acknowledgment of this boundary, so the mycelium just keeps directly on growing, and because it has no place else to go, it just grows over itself, creating overlay.

By setting the freshly cased substrate under lights immediately, misting normally, permitting sufficient ventilation, and taking care not to overheat your growing area, the culture will fruit when it is ready, and overlay won't occur.

Scratching

When the casing layer is applied, it is ideal to avoid touching or manipulating it, so you don't harm the delicate primordia or present contaminants. Be that as it may, in spite of your earnest attempts, there may in any case be events when you experience overlay. Provided that this is true, you can safeguard a casing layer by scratching it. To scratch a casing layer, simply take a clean metal fork, sterilize it with scouring alcohol, and tenderly scratch the casing down to the top of the substrate layer (make an effort not to touch the casing with your hands as you do as such). Extricate it up however much as could be expected, while maintaining an even depth.

Mist the scratched casing lightly and permit it to hatch in your fruiting chamber as in the past. In the event that you are scratching more than one container, always sterilize your fork after everyone to avoid spreading concealed contaminants. The mycelium in more established overlaid casings is potentially already dead and conveys a higher likelihood of contamination. Along these lines, this method is best when done as ahead of schedule as conceivable after the issue is discovered.

Contamination

While casing soils themselves are generally resistant to contamination, the mycelium itself is less along these lines, especially as its ages. Typically, contamination sets in simply after a few flushes of mushrooms have been harvested and the substrate is almost depleted of supplements. If contamination occurs from the get-go in the casing stage, it is most likely a sign of an issue inhabitant in the substrate or the casing soil itself, and the culture is best discarded for starting with a clean one.

As somewhere else, endeavoring to "spare" a polluted culture is generally not worth the disappointment, and is just likely to spread the contamination to different containers. There is one type of contamination remarkable to casing soils that you may every so often experience. This is Dactylium dendroides, also called "cobweb mold," for its wispy, web-like appearance. It begins as small pinpoints of fine, white fluff on top of the casing layer, and rapidly grows to cover it completely. Cobweb mold is handily spread between containers at the slightest air unsettling influence, so debased cultures ought to be removed when they are discovered. Whenever permitted to proliferate, it will eventually assault and overview any mushrooms or primordia in the container, decreasing them to a vile mush.

Once in a while beginning growers will mistake the underlying growth of mushroom mycelium into the casing layer for cobweb mold. Genuine cobweb mold grows as a fluffy layer on top of the casing soil, while the mushroom mycelium rises through it from underneath. In addition, mushroom mycelium, while it might look wispy from the outset, will immediately thicken in appearance. The occurrence of cobweb mold can be prevented by maintaining satisfactory air exchange inside the fruiting container, avoiding over the top humidity levels, and purifying the casing soil preceding application.

CHAPTER 8

Fruiting and harvesting

Many other cultivated species of mushrooms need a drop in temperature or an expansion in humidity to improve fruiting, but P cubensis does not. Thanks to a humid environment, appropriate exchange of gas, and ample light, P cubensis can yield precipitous fruit, often before the mycelium has penetrated the surface of the case layer. A variety of growers suggest extensive misting or fanning systems and cold stunning the crop by freezing it in a refrigerator overnight to start fruiting, but we consider these methods superfluous. Because the strain being cultivated is a fiery fruit tree and its essential requirements have been met, it should survive.

In this way, your efforts are best spent on discovering a good fruiting strain at a timely time, as opposed to working hard to get a poor one to fruit. In case you are familiar with the "PF Tek," you should already find much of this section commonplace. You should see primordia, little mushrooms at their most immature stage, starting to form in a few days to about fourteen days after casing. Ideally, they will grow inside the casing layer and will not be visible until smaller than expected mushrooms are already shaped all around. They tend to grow incredibly fast when they have accomplished this size (around 1 h cm) and may seem to arrive practically overnight at full size. As they grow, water will be drawn from the secret substratum and casing layer, so make sure that misting increases differently (always taking care not to overwater).

Harvesting

When the mushroom has arrived at a fitting size for productive spore dispersal (for the most part somewhere close to 3 inches and 6 inches in tallness), it stops growing and its cap augments, opening to expose its gills to the atmosphere. The best time to harvest your mushrooms is only before this point, when the veil is stretched however not broken, since after this point the mushrooms will never again put on any real weight. In addition, you don't need spores falling onto your casing soil and containers.

Given the cosmic numbers of spores produced by a solitary mushroom, this can make a serious chaos; in addition, the gases discharged by sprouting spores can potentially hinder further fruiting. The easiest way to tell when a mushroom is preparing to open is to give close consideration to the partial veil, the thin protective film that covers the gills. At first, the cap is completely enrolled (looking a lot of like those good old globe-on-a-shaft streetlamps), and the partial veil is covered up. As the cap starts to expand, the veil develops as a roundabout, light-colored band around the bottom hemisphere of the cap.

When the cap begins to flatten out, the partial veil gets stretched past its ability to expand and begins to tear, pulling away from the outer edges of the gills. Eventually, the partial veil separates from the cap entirely and its leftovers stay joined to the stipe in a skirt-like ring, known as an annulus.

Ideally, you need to pick your mushrooms when the partial veil is visible, or at the latest, when the veil begins to break. Harvesting the mushrooms is as basic as getting a handle on them at the base and bending tenderly while pulling up into the clouds from the casing. Any piece of the mushroom that remaining parts in the casing will rot, so take care to remove everything, down to the base of the stipe, utilizing forceps or a pair of clean chopsticks if fundamental. Do whatever it takes not to touch the casing layer legitimately with your hands and take extraordinary care not to harm less-created mushrooms or primordia close by.

Sometimes, it is difficult to avoid upsetting or evacuating close by mushrooms when harvesting. Right now, is smarter to remove these "babies" as well, instead of leaving them behind. Upsetting them often cuts off their association with the substrate and they stop growing and eventually rot. Don't stress a lot over the periodic loss, since whatever vitality the culture would have expended on these fruits will be occupied to the following flush. Generally, a considerable lot of vermiculite will be adhered to the base of the harvested mushrooms, leaving behind a divot in the casing layer. When you are done harvesting, simply fill these holes with fresh, appropriately moistened casing soil, mist altogether, and return the container to the fruiting area.

During the period immediately following a harvest, increment misting recurrence and quantity essentially, so as to replace the substantial amount of water removed from the casing in the harvested mushrooms. Every container should produce three to five harvests, or flushes, of mushrooms with a week or so of recovery time between each flush.

Generally, the initial barely any flushes are the most plenteous. After the fourth or fifth flush, the substrate will be exhausted, the mass of substrate will have noticeably shrunk, and the number of mushrooms that form will be insignificant. Now, the containers ought to be discarded, since the mycelium in them will begin to kick the bucket. Weak or dead mycelium is likely to get debased with molds, which could then spread to your healthy cultures.

Cleaning the Harvest

Over the long haul, it is simpler and much better hoping to clean off the mushroom stems when they are fresh as opposed to after they have been dried. Any casing soil staying on the base of harvested mushrooms can be removed by delicately scratching it off with a blade in a descending movement.

Yields and Biological Efficiency

Exactly what number of mushrooms would it be a good idea for you to hope to harvest from a specific amount of substrate? To address this inquiry, we have to allude to the idea of Biological Efficiency, or B.E., a term created by the business mushroom industry. The biological efficiency of a mushroom is its characteristic ability to change over substrate into mushrooms; A B.E. of 1 00% means either a 25% change of the wet mass of the substrate into fresh mushrooms, or a 1 0% transformation of the dry substrate into dry mushrooms. At the end of the day, at 1 00% B.E., 1 00 g dry wheat berries could be relied upon to produce around 1 00 g fresh mushrooms, or 1 0 9 dries.

P cubensis is a genuinely vigorous species, and commonly accomplishes yields a lot higher than 1 00% B.E. (maybe as much as 200%, or a 20 g for every 1 00 g dry substrate). Notwithstanding, it is generally recommended that you not have a go at extracting each and every mushroom from your containers, and instead start fresh ones. As a rule, after the third or fourth flush the number of fruits produced will greatly decay and the culture will get vulnerable to contamination, which could then handily spread to healthy cultures close by.

After the Harvest

Preserving Mushrooms

You can store fresh mushrooms in the refrigerator for up to seven days, without rotting or losing power. For example, they should be put in a breathable container, a paper (not plastic) bag, or a sealable plastic container fastened with a paper towel, slightly ajar to the lid. If you need to store your mushrooms for longer periods, you can maintain them in one way or another, as psilocybin and its related mixtures oxidize easily and become inactive when exposed to the atmosphere. The easiest and best preservation tool is to dry out. Dry psilocybin mushrooms, kept from light, heat, and moisture, can maintain their potency for a long, even years. Gradually drying the fresh mushrooms under gentle heat (1 10 ° F or below) until the "cracker" is firm, and no longer supple. Then put them, for example, in a sealed container, a zippered cooler bag or, even better, a heat-sealed bag for storing food.

Before sealing it, however much air as required should be expelled from the container. Singular bags should be put in an optional sealed container for added protection before freezing. If space is at a premium, after drying, the mushrooms may be powdered in a zest plant or coffee processor, but they will not maintain their potency as long as they are kept intact, because their chemical components will be exposed to the atmosphere for a greater amount. A kitchen food dehydrator makes an excellent drying apparatus for mushrooms, especially one that has accurate temperature control and a circulating ventilator. The best models circle warm air in a flat way which results in all racks being dried. By building a wooden box with removable, sliding wire screen racks and an I SO-watt radiant light bulb at its base as a heat source, a makeshift food dehydrator can also be handy designed. On the other hand, mushrooms may be dried by putting them over a radiator overnight in a warm oven or on a rack. Make sure to use gentle heat, 110 ° F (4Y C) or underneath, whatever drying system you use. At higher temperatures dried mushrooms will be harsh tasting and substantially less active.

Spore Printing

Freshly harvested mushrooms being stacked into a food dehydrator. Spore printing, like tissue cloning, is a method of preserving the hereditary makeup of your cultures. Spores are the result of sexual propagation, which means that a spore print will contain a wide range of genotypes. As in human propagation, every individual spore (or "child") will be made from some irregular blend of characters from every one of its two parent cores. Carefully, a spore print will never contain the very same hereditary qualities as the mushroom it originated from (unlike tissue cloning, which will).

By the by, Psilocybe mushroom species are regularly very steady starting with one age then onto the next, and the great greater part of spores in a print will behave indistinguishably from their parents. Spore prints can remain viable for quite a long time if they are kept from light, heat, and moisture. In this way, they represent a form of protection in case a cloned strain loses life or is lost through and through.

Making a Spore Print

1. To take a spore print, you will require a mushroom on which the cap is flat, and the gills are fully opened. (This is the one example when you should let the mushroom create past the globe-on-a-stick organize and permit the partial veil to begin to break before harvesting.) As with cloning, pick just the largest, most powerful specimens for spore printing, and make multiple prints at whatever point conceivable.

2. With a clean, sharp blade, cut the stem of the mushroom just beneath where it connects to the cap, so when placed face down, it will be raised a millimeter or two over the printing surface. Make the cut as clean and flat as conceivable so as to give a level and stable base. With the tip of the blade, remove any hints of the partial veil from the gills. Avoid touching the gills straightforwardly.

3. Prints can be developed on paper, glass microscope slides, or aluminum foil. Of these, glass or foil are ideal, because they can be sterilized by cleaning them down

with alcohol and drying before use, and their smooth surface texture permits the spores to be effortlessly removed with an inoculation loop later on. Clean plastic Petri dishes work pleasantly also, gave the cap is sufficiently small to fit serenely within them. Take a few prints on a solitary sheet of foil, leaving abundant space I between each cap, with the goal that the foil can be collapsed over e print for capacity. I f utilizing slides, you will most likely need to use a few to contain an entire cap.

4. Sterilize the printing surface with alcohol and permit to dry.

5. Place the cap face down on the printing material and cover it with a transformed container to maintain a humid environment and limit air flows.

6. Within a couple of hours, the cap ought to have stored its print onto the foil. Slower delivering specimens can be left overnight to create a denser print, if fundamental.

7. The finished print ought to be sealed to limit contamination. In the event that utilizing foil or paper, cut out the print, and crease clean foil over it, taking care not to press directly on the spores beneath. Seal the edges by collapsing them over. If you use glass microscope slides, cover the print with a clean blank slide, and tape the edges.

8. Place the prints inside zippered stockpiling bags and imprint them with the date and some other important information. Spore prints ought to be stored in a detect that is away from light, moisture, and heat, however, ought not be refrigerated or solidified. All around preserved spore prints can remain viable for a long time.

CHAPTER 9
Outdoor cultivation

Outside mushroom cultivation offers a number of important advantages over growing inside. When an outside garden bed has bet1n set up, it will fruit every year for quite a while, until the substrate has been fully consumed. By intermittently adding fresh wood chips to the mixture, or by creating another bed close by and utilizing a portion of the first substrate as inoculum, the life of a bed can be extended uncertainly. Such beds require practically no maintenance past keeping them damp during the drier, hotter months of the mid-year. Since wood chips are modest, and can even sometimes be had for free, outside cultivation is economical.

Wood based substrates are far less inclined to colonization by bacteria and molds, so they can be handled openly, unafraid of contamination. Finally, since they can be handily incorporated into pretty much any obscure, off the beaten path garden area, outside mushroom gardens are definitely more discreet and low profile than some other mushroom cultivation method. In spite of the fact that the substrate colonization and fruiting stages of open-air cultivation require next to no maintenance, the early stages are pretty much indistinguishable from those required for P cubensis cultivation. Spores are developed utilizing the cardboard plate method, and the subsequent mycelium is grown out on agar in Petri dishes, and afterward transferred to sterile grain. When the grain spawn is fully colonized, it is used to immunize small quantities of sterilized wood-based substrate. This wood-based spawn is used to immunize a large quantity of wood chips, which are then utilized to create the last bed. When the fruiting substrate is fully colonized, fruitings initiate when the surrounding temperatures fall into the 40° F range, from mid-October until early winter in northern North America. Flushes show up once at regular intervals or something like that, as long as temperature remains consistent.

Temperature Requirements

P cubensis and the different lignicolous (wood loving) Psilocybes will fruit outside just if your nearby temperatures drop into the forties every harvest time and stay there for a few weeks or more. In the event that you live in Florida or southern California, you will sadly need to adhere to growing P cubensis) or think about moving some place less soothing.

About Wood Substrates

The mycelium of the "wood-loving" species will grow readily on pretty much anything derived from trees, inasmuch as it is either made from hardwoods, or derived from softwoods that have been stripped of their aromatic constituents, like most paper items. With regards to fruiting, they are progressively specific, and will just do as such from a mixture of hardwood chips and sawdust.

In any case, you have a wide variety of substrate alternatives with regards to the pre-fruiting stages of cultivation. Wood-based substrates are naturally resistant to attack by molds and bacteria, so they need not be sterilized before use. Substrates that are readily consumed by certain fungi, while resistant to attack by different organisms, are known as specific for those species. Wood is basically made out of cellulose and lignin. Lignin particles are long, cross-linked chains of phenolic natural mixes. The bonds that make up lignin are incredibly chemically steady, which gives wood its trademark hardness and longevity. As a log consuming in your fireplace will affirm, there is a great arrangement of vitality contained in wood, yet it is bound firmly within the lignin latticework and isn't effortlessly gotten to by most organisms. In fact, the main organisms that can break down and expend lignin are sure species of fungi.

The fungi that have the fundamental proteins to do so are called "lignicolous" or "wood-possessing" fungi, a gathering that incorporates the caramel-cap Psilocybes. The selectivity of wood substrates for lignicolous fungi is the thing that makes them extensively simpler to handle than materials like grain. One intriguing feature of these species is that cultures gathered from the wild or from healthy cultivated beds are amazingly versatile, capable of flourishing under conditions that "virgin" pure spawn cultures would not survive. This is because introduction to different difficulties invigorates a living being to express its full capabilities.

Virgin cultures that have grown distinctly on sterile media made of straightforward components have not very many of their chemical creating qualities actuated. Free-living organisms, then again, have needed to contend day by day with a wide range of different species, and have by need built up the capacity to survive in their presence. Such "acclimated" cultures assembled from the wild are shockingly hearty.

They will grow readily on unsterilized substrates, and often appear to improve on "dirty" substrates than on clean ones. Obviously, in the event that you are starting from a spore print, this fact will be of little use to you, in any event from the outset. You despite everything need to use sterile methods in the early stages of the procedure: from cardboard plates to agar, at that point to grain, lastly to sterilized wood. Be that as it may, in the event that you are lucky to approach an already settled bed, either because you live where these mushrooms grow in the wild, or because you or somebody you know experiences already gone to the difficulty of creating one, you can do without clean methods out and out, and simply transfer mycelium to fresh substrate to create another bed.

CHAPTER 10

The chemistry of Psilocybe mushrooms

The chemical compounds present in Psilocybe mushrooms are a group of similar tryptamines, substances consisting of an indole ring and an amine bound to a two-carbon chain. If in this chapter you find the actual chemistry a little esoteric, don't stress too much. The essential take-away lesson is this: these compounds are all closely related to the natural amino acid L-tryptophan from which they are produced by the fungus, and to serotonin (5-hydroxytryptamine), a major mammalian neurotransmitter that helps to explain their pharmacological effects on humans.] Psilocin and its phosphate ester psilocybin are the most common compounds found in these fungi, while bae Psilocybin is quickly converted into psilocin by eliminating its phosphate group in the body, making the two compounds more or less identical in effects and potency after their different molecular weights are taken into consideration. The psychoactive effects of baeocystin and norbaeocystin in isolation are not well understood but there is some evidence to suggest modulating the psychoactive effects of psilocybin and psilocybin. Their existence in varying amounts may help explain common anecdotal reports of subjective differences from one species of Psilocybe mushroom to another. In the first place, almost nothing definitive is known about why these chemicals are present in those mushrooms, due to the various legal barriers to public scientific study of these mushroom species.

Nature seldom does anything without a practical purpose, especially when the action is energetically expensive, as it is here for sure. Such compounds have to serve some evolutionary advantage for the survival of these species; otherwise, for example, the resources which go into synthesizing them would be better spent on making more spores or larger fruit bodies. One might be tempted to suggest that these molecules guarantee the mushroom species ' survival because their existence allows people to grow and spread them for their psychoactive effects. Such logic, however, gives human beings far more credit than they owe, as these fungi just got along fine tor millions of years without our help. During their constant struggle to compete and survive in the natural environment, the chemicals they produce must have had a certain important purpose. Many organisms produce chemicals in their environment which have some positive or negative ecological effects on other species. Such compounds are often referred to as "secondary" metabolites, since they are not known to have any primary effect on the internal functioning of the organism itself, but are better considered as allochemicals, compounds whose effect is intended to influence other organisms. Allelochemicals can serve three roles that are interrelated: semiotic, competitive and/or symbiotic. Semiotic compounds give the receiver a signal to come closer or stay away. Many flowers ' powerful scents are meant to attract pollinating insects or animals, while other organisms discourage foraging from the bitter compounds in other plant leaves. Competitive chemicals can be defensive or offensive at once, or both.

A honeybee's sting does no lasting harm to its victim, but it does all the same teach a valuable lesson in avoidance. On the other hand, that of the hornet or wasp aims primarily at killing its insect prey. Symbiotic allochemicals give both producer and recipient mutual benefit: the Colibri receives nourishing nectar in exchange for (unwittingly) pollen spreading from one flower to another. It is not known what allochemicals function psilocybin might serve for the fungi which produce it, but it is most likely defensive. It can help prevent other organisms from competing for resources or feeding on the tender and nutrient-rich hyphae while exploring the substrate environment. Maybe these chemicals kill or inhibit the growth of snails, slugs, or worms.] They may also possess antibiotic properties, helping prevent bacteria or other fungi from attacking the fungus.

The fact that they are produced in a lot greater concentrations in the fruit bodies than in the bare mycelium lends support to the possibility that they serve a cautious capacity: if the objective of the mushroom life cycle is to produce and discharge whatever number spores as could reasonably be expected, the fruits require the greatest protection from attack. Regardless of whether these molecules are not synthesized by the fungus for the "purpose" of empowering a progressing relationship with human creatures, there is no doubt that they do effetely affect the human brain. It could be contended that these effects are unplanned, yet not circumstantial: human creatures developed in a similar environment as worms, bacteria, and fungi, and are made up from a similar fundamental chemical and biological structure blocks. Numerous organisms have tryptamine-like molecules in them; however, they are firmly related chemically, the capacities they serve are often as various as the organisms themselves. Researcher like to use the lock-and-key metaphor to depict the activity of chemicals on biological systems: when the key (the chemical) is embedded into the lock (the receptors on or inside the cells of the living being), some effect occurs. Because all organisms advanced from a typical progenitor, the number of such chemical "keys" is constrained, while their effects are most certainly not. What happens when you put psilocybin into a slug or into a human depends upon the area and the capacity of the receptors with which it associates. Precisely how psilocybin produces the effects that it does on the human brain is still particularly a puzzle, both because of the profound intricacy of the organ and the legal limitations placed on the study of psychedelic molecules. By the by, it is believed that its essential effect is mostly the consequence of its cooperation with certain serotonin receptors.

Neurobiologists allude to two nonexclusive types of dynamic molecules: agonists and foes. An agonist ties to a receptor with a similar effect as the real neurotransmitter, while an adversary blocks the effect of the neurotransmitter. Coming back to our lock-and-key metaphor, an agonist is a key that fits and turns the lock, however maybe with pretty much efficiency than the neurotransmitter itself, while a rival only sticks in the lock, preventing the real key from getting in. Psilocybin and related molecules are thought to be serotonin agonists. They tie to receptors and follow up on them much like serotonin does, yet with a slightly extraordinary proclivity. While the effect at every individual receptor site may be inconspicuous, their general effect on the human mind is obviously profound.

Psilocybin Safety Given their powerful psychological effects on humans and their theoretical functions as defensive allochemicals, one might reasonably wonder if the compounds found in Psilocybe mushrooms could be toxic to human health in any way. There is in fact no evidence to suggest they are poisonous at all. First of all, they are unlikely to be toxic, as they have such a long history of human use with no single death attributed. Moreover, these molecules were subjected to traditional toxicology tests many times, which proved to be quite innocuous.

Psilocybin has an LD-50(or 50 percent lethal dose) of about 250mg / kg in rats and mice, which means you need to give 250 milligrams of psilocybin to the test animals for every kilogram of body weight to kill half of them. Approximately, what this means for humans is that the average adult SO-kilogram male would need to ingest 22 grams of pure psilocybin, or about 500 grams of dried Psilocybe cubensis mushrooms, to earn a 50 percent chance of dying! By comparison, caffeine, widely considered a benign human drug, has an LD-50 of 1 92mg / kg in rats, making it as "toxic" as psilocybin about 1-5 times.

CHAPTER 11

The Psilocybe mushroom experience

We assume that you would not experience gone to all the difficulty to figure out how to grow psilocybin-containing mushrooms without some previous direct experience with their psychoactive effects, and some comprehension on the most proficient method to use them. In the event that you are curious about their effects, we conm1end your excitement and assurance for having come this far on the unimportant guarantee of the delights and ponders that these mushrooms can uncover. We assume that before you push off onto these huge, still generally strange, and always secretive waters, you will have done your homework.

Counsel with other people who have gone before you, either in person, on the web, or in print.! The more you know before you set off, the better prepared you will be for the secrets you will experience, and the more fortunes you will have the option to convey with you on your arrival. We have a couple of recommendations for how to make the greater part of the mushroom experience. Obviously, you should think about such exhortation while taking other factors into consideration since, as always, your mileage may shift.

Fresh versus Dry

Since all things considered, your cultivation undertakings will give definitely a greater number of mushrooms than you might require at any one time, you will likely dry them for long-term stockpiling and sometime in the future. Psilocybe mushrooms can be ingested fresh, however there are two factors to consider if you choose to do as such. To begin with, fresh mushrooms are approximately 90% water by weight, so you should multiply the weight of your dosage by a factor of 10 when utilizing fresh mushrooms.

In addition, numerous people (your modest creators included) find fresh mushrooms impressively less edible than dried ones for some unknown explanation. More than once have we eaten freshly picked mushrooms to find ourselves affiicted with issues, heartburn, and general discomfort for a great part of the journey. Drying them appears to dispose of whatever factor produces these effects. One way to avoid acid reflux when utilizing fresh mushrooms is to make an implantation from them (as described underneath) and discard the solids in the wake of soaking. In the event that you do choose to eat fresh specimens, make sure they are clean, firm, and as of late picked. More established, delicate fruits can harbor bacteria and ought to be discarded.

Dosage

Recommending a dosage system for mushroom ingestion is convoluted by the great variability in the potency of mushrooms, both among various species, and between strains or flushes of similar species. In addition to the great variety in potency among various mushrooms, there is likewise an undeniable and often wide variety in individual sensitivity to psilocybin. What may be a threshold dose (at the end of the day, the most reduced conceivable amount expected to feel any effect at all) for one person might be a whopper for another. It is very important that every person be all around familiar with their own sensitivity before exploring different avenues regarding a new example or dosage. If all else fails, it is always best to decide in favor of alert; you can always take increasingly next time around, or much later on, after the effects of the primary dose have made themselves fully felt. (An hour and a half is typically adequately long to hold up before taking a supporter dose.) One important influence on individual sensitivity is body mass; because the drug is distributed pretty much uniformly all through the body after ingestion, a heavier person will require a larger dose to accomplish a similar effect as somebody of small stature. Thus, recommended dosages of pure mixes are given as milligrams per kilogram of body mass (mg per kg). One kilogram is equal to 2.2 pounds.

Dosage levels
Low Dose: 5-1 0 mg alkaloids

At this level, the mushrooms have quite recently started to make themselves felt, creating a gentle, indistinct adjusted state, not unlike an "up" marijuana high. The body feels stimulated and the mind alert. Senses and perceptions are heightened. Colors may appear to be more splendid and progressively striking, music and sounds often appear to be increasingly particular and fresh, tastes are enhanced, etc.

While perceptions of the outer world are lightly adjusted, genuine sound or visual hallucinations are unlikely to occur at this dosage. Such low doses are agreeable to use in open settings, for example, workmanship museums or musical shows, since one's outward appearance will be sufficiently ordinary to avoid pulling in undesirable attention from strangers. This is likewise an excellent dose level for daytime investigation and contemplatory' of the natural world. £ The effects at this level generally commence within 30 minutes, and last from 2-4 hours.

Medium Dose: 1 2-25 mg alkaloids

At this level, both shut and open-peered toward visual hallucinations can emerge. At first, and at the lower range of the medium dosage, these are basically exceptionally colored, striking geometric examples, not unlike elaborate, living Oriental mats. Synesthesis, where at least two senses cross or cover are normal at this level. Tastes, smells, touch, music and different sounds can enhance and synergize with the visuals in amazing and astounding ways, and the other way around. At slightly higher doses, conceptual dreams can give way to progressively pictorial images, both recognizable and strange. With adequate experience and solace with these dosage levels, one can wander out into the natural world, to great effect, yet we recommend avoiding contact with strangers at whatever point conceivable. The effects at this level generally starts within 30 minutes, and last from 3-5 hours.

High Dose: 30-40 mg alkaloids

At these doses, the sky really is the limit. Terence McKenna alluded to such amounts as "chivalrous doses," since each experience is definitely a journey into uncharted waters. What you will find we can't state, since the experience will be exceptionally personal and always particular. We do anyway recommend that you make sure to find yourself in agreeable and protected settings before you begin, free from interruptions and undesirable shocks. Quiet darkness, alone or with a guide is ideal for such voyages. Don't think about wandering out into the "real world" at this dose level. You presumably won't have the option to stand up, considerably less stroll with any amount of coordination anyway. At high doses, the mushroom experience generally commences within 30 minutes, and endures from 5-7 hours.

Higher Doses

We don't recommend doses much past 0.5mg/kg, in any event, for the most experienced and valiant explorer. After this point the theory of consistent losses sets in, and the experience turns out to be longer and progressively intense without fundamentally being all the more fulfilling. Psilocybe alkaloids are very benevolent to human health and it is basically difficult to take an "overdose," at any rate one that is truly harmful to human health. In the event that you find you have taken more than you ought to have, coincidentally or something else, have confidence that, in spite of the intensity of the experience, you will most likely survive. Indeed, even at very high doses, the experience will last no longer than 8 hours, with the most intense part over far sooner than that.

Monoamine Oxidase (MAO) Inhibitors and Psilocybe Alkaloids

If you are as of now taking monoamine oxidase medications of any kind, you ought not to ingest psilocybin (or any psychedelics, for that matter.) These drugs are intended to deactivate the human chemical system answerable for the digestion of numerous drugs and basic food poisons. With MAO idle, aggravates the body would somehow or another corrupt can have unpredictable and potentially perilous effects. In the event that you are taking MAO inhibitors for depression (their most basic sign), you should hold up until you have stopped taking them before exploring different avenues regarding psilocybin. Another psychedelic, the Amazonian blend ayahuasca, deliberately joins a MAO inhibitor from the vine Bannisteriopsis caapi with a tryptamine-containing plant to produce its effects. Some smart "psychonauts" have used this model to create a "mycohuasca" by joining Psilocybemushrooms with B. caapi or other MAO-repressing plants, dramatically potentiating and adjusting their effects. We don't recommend doing as such, however in the event that you choose to try different things with something like this yourself, it would be ideal if you be careful and, as always, get your work done.

Tolerance

At the point when psilocybin is used more than once every week, tolerance generally occurs. The specific causes behind this phenomenon are not surely known, yet the general effect is that the brain turns out to be incidentally desensitized to a specific drug after every presentation. While tolerance to psilocybin can be overwhelmed by essentially expanding the dose, it is ideal to simply hold up at any rate a week between voyages to give the brain (just as your mind) a chance to come back to baseline.

Methods of ingestion

A great many people simply bite and swallow the dried mushrooms. For the individuals who find them to some degree not exactly agreeable, it is simple enough to make an extract, since the alkaloids in Psilocybe mushrooms are freely dissolvable in both ethanol and hot water. Regardless of what method of ingestion you use, it is prudent to wait for a least 6 hours before utilizing Psilocybe mushrooms, to minimize heartburn and to expand retention of the alkaloids.

Mushroom Tea

Simply make a pot of your preferred home-grown tea utilizing one and one-half cups of water per person, preferably utilizing aromatic herbs and flavors, for example, mint, cinnamon, or cloves to help cover the taste of the mushrooms and to quiet the stomach. In the wake of soaking the tea for 10 minutes or somewhere in the vicinity, pour it into a subsequent pot containing the imperative amount of fresh or dried mushrooms. Cover this and permit to soak for in any event one hour, mixing every so often. Strain and pour into the suitable number of teacups. The remaining mushroom solids might be eaten, yet this is generally redundant, since the vast majority of the alkaloids will have infused into the tea. High temperatures will quickly corrupt alkaloids, so the soaking fluid ought to never be permitted to boil once the mushrooms have been added. If the tea isn't used immediately, it ought to be refrigerated. When prepared, mushroom tea ought to be used within 48 hours.

Alcohol Extract

For a longer enduring preparation, think about making an extract. Squashed or powdered mushrooms can be soaked in high-proof alcohol (1 50-proof or greater, for example, rum or Ever clear, utilizing 25-50 milliliters of alcohol for each dose. Subsequent to soaking for 3 days or longer, the extract can be filtered or tapped and stored for a while or longer without extensive loss of potency.

CHAPTER 12

How to grow your own psychedelic mushrooms

It is recommended to build your own fungi culture at home in case you need to be separate from the cache of fungi out in nature and the contributions from some smart shops in specific countries. There are different cultivation methods for each specie. The most cultivated psychedelic mushrooms are Psilocybe cubensis, sometimes called the "Mexican." The reason they are so popular is because under controlled conditions, they are very easy to grow. In Europe they have to be grown indoors. Then again there are various species that can grow outside effectively. Psilocybe cyanescens are local fungi that grow similarly on wood chips as does the Psilocybe azurescens. The methods of cultivating the two last once, however, are very special to the technique for growing Psilocybe cubensis.

In general, it's a little harder to grow your own fungi than cultivating your own weed. Before you start with the culture of the fungi you have to learn basic concepts and function precisely. The biggest problem is job sterile more often than not. If one starts planting, you know very quickly that crops of fungi are susceptible to bacteria and mold. Whether you are really working properly and sterilizing your glass with the culture can get infected even now. Don't get distracted by the boy! Observe just what you are doing and what has turned out badly. Attempt to make a profit from your mistake.

Guidance to cultivate your own fungi Source:

The following technique was distributed without precedent for Seattle in September 1991 under the name PF TEK (Psilocybe Fanaticus technique). Around 1998 the greater part a million of models were available for use. The PF TEK is the most famous natural fungi grow technique in the world. This approved variant was adjusted to circumstance in Europe by the Stitching Perfect Fungi.

One needs the following extras:

- ✓ Drug store
- ✓ Needles with needle protection
- ✓ Clean packed infusion needles
- ✓ Syringes and needles are just important when one needs to make its own spore's syringes
- ✓ Development market or hardware store
- ✓ Awl (or knitting needle)
- ✓ Drugstore
- ✓ Spiritus (70–80% volume alcohol)
- ✓ Small and bended line cuticle scissors or small scissors with small tip
- ✓ Antibacterial cleanser
- ✓ Spongy cotton
- ✓ Gardening shop
- ✓ Plant sprayer
- ✓ Perlit
- ✓ Vermikulit (corn size 0–3mm, grade nr. 2)
- ✓ Household article (market, store, health shop, etc)
- ✓ Tinfoil
- ✓ Autoclave
- ✓ Lighter

- ✓ Glasses with smooth sidewalls
- ✓ 15 watts-bulb
- ✓ Purple bug lamp or 370-nm-black light (Philips color 5)
- ✓ Kitchen fork
- ✓ Cooler
- ✓ Beaker
- ✓ Estimating scoop
- ✓ Translucent plastic bag
- ✓ Rice flour or brown rice
- ✓ Soup bowl
- ✓ Toilette paper
- ✓ Stationery shop
- ✓ Elastic groups
- ✓ Marker
- ✓ Sellotape
- ✓ Pressing film
- ✓ Pet shop
- ✓ Smaller than expected aquarium
- ✓ Thermometer for the aquarium

Besides, one ought to have a residue free room (for instance a big material closet or a not particularly used shower), a scratch plate, a seating convenience, a blowtorch and a cooler with freezers.

1 — Glasses

Deal with the surface of the glasses when you're picking. Along these lines, you'll have a substantially more open to harvesting process. More smaller glasses are superior to a ton of big size glasses. The reason accordingly is that there will happen contaminations occasionally.

1.1 One takes:

Appropriate glasses which are easy to upset like a cake tin. The glasses must not deform during the process of cooking out.

1.2 Glasses which were already used a couple of times

Reasonable glasses made out of white glass are jelly glasses up to 385 ml or preserving jars.

1.3 Plastic glasses and form

Sterilisable jars made out of heat-resistant plastic, for example, Polypropylene (PP) are functional. The name is often discovered in a small triangular image. They're modest, light and unbreakable, yet not offer handy to close.

1.4 Drinking glasses

Drinking glasses are additionally alright for cultivating. At the point when you use those as a tank, you'll use the tinfoil as a cover. When utilizing them there's a bigger chance of getting infected than when you're utilizing glasses with a screw-cap. At the point when you fix the foil with an elastic band and take a thicker layer of Vermiculite you can limit the risk.

2 Preparation of the soil and the process of sterilize

Fungi are more easy organisms than plants. They do not need any chlorophyll and along these lines acquire oxygen just as azotic from outside.

2.1.1 One takes:

Rice flour or brown rice (self-processed brown rice is superior to pre-packed rice flour)

- ✓ Medium coarse Vermiculite
- ✓ Glasses with smooth sidewalls
- ✓ Beaker
- ✓ Sellotape
- ✓ Awl or knitting needle
- ✓ Soup bowl
- ✓ Kitchen fork

2.1.2 Recipe for the preparation of the soil

A most extreme harvest will be accomplished when you use a 1/4 glass with brown rice flour, a 1/2 glass with medium coarse Vermiculite and a 1/4 glass with water.

2.2 Procedure for 320 ml glasses

If you use glasses with a plastic cover (or foil covered glasses) start with stage 3.

Screw the cover on the glass.

Sting four holes into the cover.

Scoop 160 ml of Vermiculite into the soup bowl.

Scoop 80 ml of rice flour over it.

Run over carefully 80 ml of water.

Mix everything appropriately until there is no dry rice flour any longer.

Mix the soil for every cultivation container individually. Along these lines, you avoid the creation of clusters.

Fill the classes freely.

Hit smoothly the bottom of the glass with your palm. Presently, shake the glass a little with the goal that the soil can spread similarly.

Clean the edge of the glass.

Presently put a little layer of dry Vermiculite over the soil.

In the event that there's any extra Vermiculite in the glass you can take it carefully out. In any case, don't press in any of it in the soil.

Stick the holes on the cover with the sellotape and make sure that potential air pockets are removed. Close the cover however not very tight.

2.3 Sterilize

In the principal period of the growth, the Myzel is truly defenseless for infections which can be caused by mold and bacteria. In the process of cooking out, the microorganisms will get slaughtered and their generation stopped.

2.3.1 One takes:

A pot with easy closable cover. At the bottom of the pot we have to have a framework which avoids that the glasses have contact with the bottom.

2.3.2 Procedure

Cook the glasses for one hour at around 100 degree Celsius. If you have a quick cooking pot you cook it for around 30 minutes at 120-degree celsius. The cover of the pot must be closed excellent. Something else, the soil will dry out. Look to it that no water interacts with the soil and take care that there's sufficient water in the pot.

2.4 Waiting time

Preserve the glasses by room temperature. Following one month the glasses need to appear to be identical and smell like short after the disinfecting. Besides, they should be a similar weight as in the past. One can free the cover a tad and smell the content if the Vermiculite stays at the ground.

In the event that there's a contamination, it makes it significantly simpler to determine its underlying foundations.

3.0 Inoculate and growth

The seeding of the spores is called immunize. Not grow through soil is likely to get infections. To avoid potential infections, utilize the following techniques:

3.1 One takes:

Inoculum (an ampulla or syringe for 10 glasses — this is for just for PF and PFE spores)

- ✓ Lighter
- ✓ Marker
- ✓ Needle
- ✓ Thermometer

3.2 Procedure

Close every window and entrance into your home (the bathrooms are perfect for this procedure). Wash everything with a combination of Spiritus and antibacterial cleanser.

(Plastic covered glass): Sit four holes in the cover with a hot needle inside the swivel. This is not important at the stage when you are using glasses for drinking. Use a four-hole cover as a guide here.

Shake the syringe with the intention that the spores scatter in the water and eliminate needle protection.

In a soot-free fire heat up the syringe tip. A switched shot glass with a drop of Spiritus out of a pipette is used for a soot-free fire. A drop absorbs the optimal amount of time, exactly.

Place a needle through an opening and let it cool down.

Take the syringe as a ring finger between the thumbs and middle-the latchkey pointer. Keep the needle to the mirror, so that the needle tip opening is clear.

During the time that the inoculum drops into the glass you need to take the finger out of the latchkey and sit tight at that point for about a second taking the needle back. In case the syringe clogs one withdraws the blockage and you dispose of it. Warning: Don't breathe into the gap!

Repeat the four to six levels until each opening is resistant. A while later, with the help of a soot-free fire, clean the needle again and put on the protection, so you can store the impenetrable syringe.

Seal a sellotape to the holes in the cover and write the date on the bottle.

If the spores in the main glass expand, vaccinate the following glass. In a month's time you can harvest along those lines for your own use. More time, space and material expense pointless, and can reduce the quality.

3.3 Sprinkling and growth

Place the glasses in a residue-free place with no sunlight within a temperature range of 15–30 degrees celsius. An excellent match for that is a cooler. You can use a lamp to sparkle from the glasses if heath is needed. Do not use heat from below as this dries the soil out. Within a week, there are small white stains rising on the Myzel, and Mycelia emerging through the soil in the second week.

4.0 Culture surroundings

When there are primordium rising up out of the soil you can remove the glass. (Be careful with not decimating the young shrooms!) Cut the parts which are not grown through with a hot blade out of the cake, so you don't get any infections. Just full grown through soils ought to be used for fructification as though this isn't the case the risk for infections is a lot higher.

4.1 Procedure

Turn over the glass and remove the cake carefully from it. If pieces are breaking of you can put it back and it will grow on once more. The cake will smell severely and remembers to the smell of harvest time leaves. Be careful in the event that it smells somewhat sharp or smelly. Remove drops with toilette paper. Ordinarily, harmed cakes do have recolors on it, yet this isn't associated with the process of disintegrate.

4.2 Culture environment

In a good culture form:

The relative humidity stays above 85%

Ventilation and temperature are effectively controllable

The cakes can be enlightened

Everything is easy to clean

4.2.1 One takes:

Small aquarium or a straightforward fruit bowl

Straightforward bag or Plexiglas table and cover

Positioned out (saturated with water) Perlit

Plant sprayer with high pressure

4.2.2 Construction and situating

If you don't mind see the drawings for the development. In a bag with just one cake, the modesty stays high, you won't get any contamination and you'll have oxygen shortage. For the pressing of a few cakes are advantages and disadvantages the specific inverse. Perlit is capillary and lets water disintegrate speedier than Vermiculite. Add the required Perlit while it is cooking. The fume will deal with the quick humidification of the form. At that point put in the small aquarium or the fruit bowl into the bag and afterward close it. Put or attach the bag into an ice chest. Attach a black light over it. Be careful and make sure that there is enough separation between the bag and the black light, so the cake won't get dried out. Neither the black light nor the bureau is really essential — you'd likewise have the option to attach the bag in a tent or at a tree.

4.3 Nebulize process

Nebulize routinely at regular intervals the air with water. The haze will add fresh oxygen and will break down azotic. Shrooms are protected against direct water drops, so you don't have to stress over that one. Excess water can be driven away through a whole on the bottom.

4.4 Light, air and temperature

Most primordien will grow in light of 370 nanometer (beautification blacklight). Shrooms will grow to the light. Be that as it may, a photo time of beyond what 12 hours can be harmful to the shrooms.

The intensity of the light isn't that important. In the event that you despite everything can peruse with this light that is sufficiently fair. Every day ventilation is recommended. Too much carbon dioxide will hinder the growth of the hut of a few shroom species. With Psilocybe cubensis this won't be a big issue, however. The shrooms are growing with at the fastest speed when you create an environment with around 30-degree celsius. In any case, they won't be that potent nor solid. From the earliest starting point of working of some shroom pre-states a temperature of 21-degree celsius is preferably.

4.5 Shrooms and malformation

The primordial shroom rises out of the small white dots which will turn into yellow little shrooms. The first ones are deformed and will stop growing in just a few days.

The tip of an infant shroom that is "outbound" will get black gray, later black and deform from round to irregular. The hut is going to fall prematurely and get particularly thick. Various malformations exist as white knobs. Before they become brittle, harvest them with a needle-malformations, are extremely powerful!

From other pre-states the customary shrooms expand. Harvesting a quarter of the weight of the wet soil is pretty much normal. There were 4 yields of up to 60 percent in excellent situations.

5.0 Inoculum raising shroom mature spores discolor the dark cake. The danger of contamination occurs during the preparation of the inoculum. So, make sure that you function properly.

5.1 One takes:

- ✓ Glass with cover made out of steal
- ✓ Foil
- ✓ Pot or oven
- ✓ Spiritus
- ✓ Suds
- ✓ Bended cuticle scissors
- ✓ Small knife
- ✓ Lighter
- ✓ Cotton fleece
- ✓ Shot glass

5.1.1 Procedure

Tinfoil to protect the glass and possibly a flexible unit. Placed the cover in a mixture of spirits and suds by then.

Put the glasses into the broiler at 150-degree celsius for about thirty minutes or cook them out in a closed oven. The glass must not have contact to the bottom in a jar.

The windows and gateways are locked. Wash the dividers and use suds / spiritus utensils.

Placed the cooled glass alongside the cake with sporulating shrooms on the right side. Place the turned cover on the right side as well. Place a rotating shot glass with some spirit (70–80 percent) on the left side of the cake. Also put the lighter by it.

Free the foil, so you can remove it from the glass with one hand.

Douse a spirit ball made of cotton. You cleanse the knife and the scissor with this.

Light on spirit at shot glass at the edge. Steam the scissor and the tip of the knife.

Sting the hut with the knife and with the scissor pick off the stem.

Do not hold your hands over the glass — pull the foil away — cut the hut out of the knife with the scissor (see drawing nr. 10) and then put it into the glass that you can open as of now.

Let the glass rest at room temperature for 4 days.

Remove a hot knife from the hut and let the spore engrave dry. For a year, that one should be storable.

5.2 Production of the inoculum

Cook a syringe and a glass of water with a hidden entire in the cover for an hour long in a pot stacked up with water. Sting an opening into the cover of the glass where the spore engrave is put away. Sterilize the needle by heating and inject a touch of cooled and sterile water over the spores. Stick the opening with the objective that it's close again and freeze the spore water. Defrost it from there on in a manner so the glass stands inclined. While doing this, manage the ice squares. The water must not contact the cover at whatever point. Make sure the glass is hermetically sealed.

5.3 Filling of the syringes

Take a pot and fill it with water. By then cook a syringe in it similarly as a glass stacked up with water which has a hidden opening in the cover. This you time for about an hour. Sterilize the needle by heating and inject a layer of cooled and sterile water into the glass with the spore water. Hold the glass inclined and pull the syringe totally. Sterilize the needle by heating again and pack the syringe water/air proof.

6.0 Harvesting and conservation

Young shrooms are better than old ones.

Note: Decide for each shroom whether you sporulate it, eat it or if you have to dispose of it. Don't store the shrooms: the fresher the shrooms are the more potent they will be.

6.1 Harvesting

Affecting substances will amass themselves in the huts of the young shrooms. At the point when the sporulating procedure begins the shrooms will lose step by step of their potency. The snapshot of harvesting for devouring is then legitimate, when the assurance fleece is opening.

6.1.1 Once takes:

- ✓ Dry hands
- ✓ Sharp knife
- ✓ Needle

6.1.2 Procedure

Reap with dry hands. Push the shroom with a pivoting improvement away from the cake. Utilize a needle for the shorter ones. Cut social occasions of adnate shrooms first and thereafter remove the stumps.

6.2 Conservation

Blue shading shows oxidation of the Psilocybin. UV light, humidity, warmth and oxygen quicken this procedure. Drying and enemies of oxidants will obstruct this particular procedure.

6.3 Drying

Drying will decrease stomach and gut distress. Dried shrooms are best for limit.

6.3.1 One takes:

- ✓ 15-watt bulb
- ✓ Thermometer
- ✓ Shirt or sheets
- ✓ Box
- ✓ Pin

6.3.2 Procedure

Cut holes in the sides of the box and place the bulb some place in it. Stretch the shirt or sheet as a shade over it and fix it.

Put the shrooms and the thermometer on it. Make sure that the temperature won't outperform 30-degree celsius. When the shrooms begin to get wrinkled remove the Vermiculite. New shrooms then can be put away impermeable and without humidity in the cooler.

CHAPTER 13

Legal status of psilocybin mushrooms

The legal status of illegal actions involving psilocybin mushrooms varies throughout the world. Under the 1971 United Nations Convention on Psychotropic Substances, psilocybin and psilocin are listed as Schedule I drugs. Schedule I drugs are defined as drugs with high potential for abuse or drugs that have no recognized medical uses. Psilocybin mushrooms, however, have had numerous medicinal and religious uses throughout history in dozens of cultures, and have significantly lower potential for abuse than other Schedule I drugs.

U.N. treaties do not regulate psilocybin mushrooms. From a letter to the Dutch Ministry of Health, dated 13 September 2001, from Herbert Schaepe, Chairman of the United Nations International Narcotics Control Board.

As you know, mushrooms containing the aforementioned substances are collected and used for their hallucinogens. As a matter of international law, under the 1971 Convention on Psychotropic Substances, no plants (natural material) containing Psilocybe and psilocybin are currently under jurisdiction. Preparations made of these plants are therefore not subject to international control and, therefore, are not subject to the articles of the 1971 Convention. Criminal cases are decided with respect to domestic law, which might otherwise provide for restrictions on psilocybin and psilocybin-containing mushrooms. Since the Board can only speak about the contours of the international drug conventions, I cannot give an opinion on the litigation at issue.

However, many countries have some level of psilocybin mushroom regulation or prohibition (for example, the US Psychotropic Substances Act, the UK Misuse of Drugs Act 1971, and the Canadian Controlled Drugs and Substances Act). The ban on psilocybin mushrooms has been criticized by the general public and by researchers who see therapeutic potential in drug addictions and other mental instabilities such as PTSD, anxiety and depression. There are also relatively few medical risks among regulated drugs, psilocybin mushrooms.

There is a lot of ambiguity about the legal status of psilocybin mushrooms in many national, state, and provincial drug laws, as well as a strong element of selective enforcement in some places, since psilocybin and psilocin are considered illegal to possess as substances without a license, but mushrooms themselves are not mentioned in those laws. The legal status of Psilocybe spores is even more ambiguous, as the spores do not contain either psilocybin or psilocin, and thus are not illegal to sell or possess in many jurisdictions, although many jurisdictions will prosecute items used in drug manufacturing under broader laws. A few jurisdictions (such as Georgia and Idaho, the US states) have specifically banned the sale and possession of psilocybin mushroom spores. Psilocybin mushroom production is considered drug manufacturing in most jurisdictions and is often heavily penalized, though some countries and one US state have ruled that growing psilocybin mushrooms do not qualify as a controlled substance "manufacturing."

Steps to Mushroom Farming

Mushroom cultivating comprises of six stages, and despite the fact that the divisions are to some degree arbitrary, these means distinguish what is expected to form a creation system.

The six stages of mushroom cultivating:

Stage I

1. Composting

Stage II

2. Composting
3. Spawning
4. Casing
5. Sticking
6. Editing

These means are described in their naturally occurring arrangement, stressing the notable features within each progression. Compost gives supplements expected to mushroom to grow. Two types of material are generally used for mushroom compost, the most used and most affordable being wheat straw-bedded horse manure. Synthetic compost is generally made from roughage and squashed corncobs, in spite of the fact that the term often alludes to any mushroom compost where the prime fixing isn't horse manure. The two types of compost require the addition of nitrogen supplements and a molding specialist, gypsum.

The preparation of compost occurs in two stages alluded to as Phase I and Phase II composting. The discussion of compost preparation and mushroom creation begins with Phase I composting.

Stage I:

1. Making Mushroom Compost

This period of compost preparation as a rule occurs outside albeit an enclosed structure or a structure with a rooftop over it might be used. A solid section, alluded to as a wharf, is needed for composting. Also, a compost turner to aerate and water the fixings, and a tractor-loader to move the fixings to the turner is required. In prior days heaps were turned by hand utilizing pitchforks, which is as yet an option in contrast to automated hardware, however it is work intensive and truly requesting.

Stage I composting is started by mixing and wetting the fixings as they are stacked in a rectangular heap with tight sides and a free center. Typically, the mass fixings are put through a compost turner. Water can be sprayed onto the horse manure or synthetic compost as these materials travel through the turner. Nitrogen enhancements and gypsum are spread over the top of the mass fixings and are completely mixed by the turner. When the heap is wetted and formed, high-impact aging (composting) commences because of the growth and multiplication of microorganisms, which occur naturally in the mass fixings. Heat, smelling salts, and carbon dioxide are discharged as side-effects during this process. Compost activators, other than those referenced, are not required, albeit some natural cultivating books pressure the requirement for an "activator."

Mushroom compost creates as the chemical idea of the raw fixings is changed over by the activity of microorganisms, heat, and some heat-discharging chemical reactions. These occasions bring about a food source generally appropriate for the growth of the mushroom to the rejection of other fungi and bacteria. There must be sufficient moisture, oxygen, nitrogen, and carbohydrates present all through the process, or else the process will stop. This is the reason water and enhancements are added occasionally, and the compost heap is aerated as it travels through the turner.

Gypsum is added to limit the oiliness compost ordinarily tends to have. Gypsum expands the flocculation of specific chemicals in the compost, and they cling to straw or roughage as opposed to filling the pores (holes) between the straws. A side advantage of this phenomenon is that air can permeate the heap all the more readily, and air is essential to the composting process. The prohibition of air results in an airless (anaerobic) environment in which pernicious chemical mixes are formed which bring down the selectivity of mushroom compost for cultivating mushrooms. Gypsum is added at the outset of composting at 40 pounds per ton of dry fixings.

Nitrogen supplements in general use today incorporate brewer's grain, seed meals of soybeans, peanuts, or cotton, and chicken manure, among others. The purpose of these enhancements is to expand the nitrogen content to 1.5 percent for horse manure or 1.7 percent for synthetic, both computed on a dry weight premise. Synthetic compost requires the addition of urea or ammonium nitrate at the outset of composting to give the compost microflora a readily accessible form of nitrogen for their growth and multiplication.

Corn cobs are sometimes inaccessible or accessible at a price considered to be unnecessary. Substitutes for or supplements to corn cobs incorporate destroyed hardwood bark, cottonseed hulls, killed grape pomace, and cocoa bean hulls. The executives of a compost heap containing any of these materials is novel in the requirements for watering and the interim between turnings.

The underlying compost heap ought to be 5 to 6 feet wide, 5 to 6 feet high, and as long as essential. A two-sided box can be used to form the heap (rick), albeit a few turners are outfitted with a "ricker", so a box isn't required. The sides of the heap ought to be firm and thick, yet the center must remain free all through Phase I composting. As the straw or feed softens during composting, the materials become less inflexible and compactions can without much of a stretch occur. If the materials become excessively conservative, air can't travel through the heap and an anaerobic environment will create.

Turning and watering are done at approximately 2-day interims, yet not except if the heap is hot (145° to 170°F). Turning gives the chance to water, aerate, and mix the fixings, just as to move the straw or feed from a cooler to a warmer area in the heap, outside versus inside. Enhancements are likewise added when the ricks are turned, however they ought to be added early in the composting process. The number of turnings and the time between turnings depends on the state of the starting material and the time fundamental for the compost to heat to temperatures above 145°F.

Steps to Mushroom Farming

Mushroom cultivating comprises of six stages, and despite the fact that the divisions are to some degree arbitrary, these means recognize what is expected to form a creation system.

The six stages of mushroom cultivating

1. Composting
2. Composting
3. Spawning
4. Casing
5. Sticking
6. Trimming

These means are described in their naturally occurring succession, accentuating the remarkable features within each progression. Compost gives supplements expected to mushroom to grow. Two types of material are generally used for mushroom compost, the most utilized and most affordable being wheat straw-bedded horse manure. Synthetic compost is generally made from feed and squashed corncobs, despite the fact that the term often alludes to any mushroom compost where the prime fixing isn't horse manure. The two types of compost require the addition of nitrogen supplements and a molding operator, gypsum.

The preparation of compost occurs in two stages alluded to as Phase I and Phase II composting. The discussion of compost preparation and mushroom creation begins with Phase I composting.

Stage I

1. Making Mushroom Compost

This period of compost preparation typically occurs outside albeit an enclosed structure or a structure with a rooftop over it might be used. A solid section, alluded to as a wharf, is required for composting. Also, a compost turner to aerate and water the fixings, and a tractor-loader to move the fixings to the turner is required. In prior days heaps were turned by hand utilizing pitchforks, which is as yet an option in contrast to automated gear, yet it is work intensive and truly requesting.

Stage I composting is started by mixing and wetting the fixings as they are stacked in a rectangular heap with tight sides and a free center. Regularly, the mass fixings are put through a compost turner. Water is sprinkled onto the horse manure or synthetic compost as these materials travel through the turner. Nitrogen enhancements and gypsum are spread over the top of the mass fixings and are completely mixed by the turner. When the heap is wetted and formed, vigorous maturation (composting) commences because of the growth and proliferation of microorganisms, which occur naturally in the mass fixings. Heat, smelling salts, and carbon dioxide are discharged as results during this process. Compost activators, other than those referenced, are not required, albeit some natural cultivating books pressure the requirement for an "activator."

Mushroom compost creates as the chemical idea of the raw fixings is changed over by the activity of microorganisms, heat, and some heat-discharging chemical reactions. These occasions bring about a food source generally appropriate for the growth of the mushroom to the rejection of other fungi and bacteria. There must be satisfactory moisture, oxygen, nitrogen, and carbohydrates present all through the process, or else the process will stop. This is the reason water and enhancements are added occasionally, and the compost heap is aerated as it travels through the turner.

Gypsum is added to limit the oiliness compost ordinarily tends to have. Gypsum expands the flocculation of specific chemicals in the compost, and they hold fast to straw or feed instead of filling the pores (holes) between the straws. A side advantage of this phenomenon is that air can permeate the heap all the more readily, and air is essential to the composting process. The rejection of air results in an airless (anaerobic) environment in which malicious chemical mixes are formed which take away from the selectivity of mushroom compost for growing mushrooms. Gypsum is included at the outset of composting at 40 lbs. per ton of dry fixings.

Nitrogen supplements in general use today incorporate brewer's grain, seed meals of soybeans, peanuts, or cotton, and chicken manure, among others. The purpose of these enhancements is to build the nitrogen content to 1.5 percent for horse manure or 1.7 percent for synthetic, both computed on a dry weight premise. Synthetic compost requires the addition of ammonium nitrate or urea at the outset of composting to give the compost microflora a readily accessible form of nitrogen for their growth and proliferation.

Corn cobs are sometimes inaccessible or accessible at a price considered to be extreme. Substitutes for or supplements to corn cobs incorporate destroyed hardwood bark, cottonseed hulls, killed grape pomace, and cocoa bean hulls. The board of a compost heap containing any of these materials is remarkable in the requirements for watering and the interim between turnings.

The underlying compost heap ought to be 5 to 6 feet wide, 5 to 6 feet high, and as long as essential. A two-sided box can be utilized to form the heap (rick), albeit a few turners are furnished with a "ricker", so a box isn't required. The sides of the heap ought to be firm and thick, yet the center must remain free all through Phase I composting. As the straw or roughage softens during composting, the materials become less inflexible and compactions can without much of a stretch occur. In the event that the materials become excessively smaller, air can't travel through the heap and an anaerobic environment will create.

Turning and watering is done at intervals of about 2 days, but not except when the heap is hot (145 ° to 170 ° F). Turning gives the opportunity to wash, aerate and mix the fixings, just as it helps the straw or feed to move from a cooler to a warmer place in the heap, outside versus inside. Equally, changes are applied when the ricks are turned, but should be added early in the composting process. The number of turns and the time between turns depends on the state of the starting material and the fundamental time to heat up to temperatures above 145 ° F for the compost.

4. Casing

The casing is a top-dressing added to the spawn-run compost that ultimately shapes the mushrooms. Clay-topsoil field soil, a combination of peat moss with calcareous earth, or weathered recycled, spent compost can be used as a casing. Casing does not need to waste time with supplements because casing is a water store and a place where rhizomorphs are produced. Rhizomorphs tend to be thick strings, which develop when the very fine mycelium fuses. Initials to the mushrooms, primordia, or pins appear on the rhizomorphs, so there will be no mushrooms without rhizomorphs. Case should be sanitized for the execution of any insects and pathogens which it may pass on. Similarly, it is important to spread the casing so that the depth is uniform over the compost surface. Such uniformity makes it possible for the spawn to pass in and through the casing at a similar rate, and eventually to produce mushrooms at the same time. Casing should have the option to retain moisture as moisture is central to a firm mushroom's growth.

Dealing with the yield in the case wake requires that the compost temperature be kept in the case wake at about 75 ° F for up to 5 days, and that the relative humidity should be high. From that point on, until small mushroom initials (pins) have grown, the compost temperature should be consistently reached down 2 ° F. Water has to be added intermittently throughout the period following the casing to raise the level of humidity to field efficiency before the mushroom pins shape. Understanding when, how and how much water to apply for casing is a "job of craftsmanship" that distinguishes seasoned growers from beginners readily.

5. Staying

Initials of the mushroom build after rhizomorphs develop in the casing. The initials on a rhizomorph are incredibly small and may be seen as outgrowths. The structure is a pin at a point where a secret quadruple in size. Through the catch arrangement pins continue to expand and grow larger, and ultimately a catch enlarges to a mushroom. Harvestable mushrooms in the wake of the casing appear to be 18 to 21 days. Pins are produced by bringing fresh air into the growing room when the carbon dioxide content of room air is reduced to 0.08 per cent or lower, depending on the cultivar. Outside air is about 0.04 percent containing carbon dioxide.

The arranging of fresh air presentation is important and is something adapted interestingly through experience. Generally, it is ideal to ventilate as small as possible until the mycelium has started to show up at the surface of the casing, and to stop watering when pin initials are forming. If the carbon dioxide is cut down too early by means of airing too soon, the mycelium stops growing through the casing and mushroom initials form beneath the surface of the casing. Everything considered mushrooms continue growing, they push through the casing and are dirty at harvest time. Too little moisture can likewise bring about mushrooms forming beneath the surface of the casing. Staying influences both the potential yield and nature of a harvest and is a colossal development in the creation cycle.

6. Trimming

The terms flush, break, or blossom are names given to the repeating 3-to 5-day harvest periods during the trimming cycle; these are followed by several days when no mushrooms are available to harvest. This cycle repeats itself in a musical way, and harvesting can go on as long as mushrooms continue maturing. Most mushroom farmers harvest for 35 to 42 days, yet some harvest a yield for 60 days, and harvest can proceed for as long as 150 days.

For good results, the air temperature should be kept between 57 ° to 62 ° F during trimming. This temperature range favors mushroom growth, but cooler temperatures will protract both disease pathogens and insect bugs from life examples. It can give the impression of being strange that there are threats that can damage mushrooms, no harvest that doesn't have to deal with different species is grown anyway. Aggravation of the mushroom can cause total yield failures, and often the critical factor in how far a harvest is dependent on the extent of infiltration of the vermin. Cultural practices combined with the use of pesticides will control these pests and insects, however it is usually appealing to exclude these species from the rising rooms.

The relative humidity in the growing rooms should be sufficiently high to limit the drying of the casing anyway not too high to cause clammy or tenacious to the cap surfaces of creating mushrooms. Water is added to the casing to prevent water pressure from producing mushrooms; this means watering 2 to 3 times a week in business practice. Every watering may include quite a lot of gallons, depending on the dryness of the wrapper, the cultivar being grown, and the time of the pins, buttons, or mushrooms going forward. The majority of first-time growers add a lot of water and the surface of the case seals; this is seen as a lack of texture on the casing sheet. Sealed case prevents the exchange of gases which are necessary for the formation of mushroom pins. One can measure how much water has been harvested after the first break by remembering that 90 per cent of the mushroom is water and a gallon of water weight 8.3 lbs. Where 100 lbs. 90 lbs of mushrooms have been picked. Water has been removed from the casing; and this is the thing to replace before the second break creates mushrooms.

Outdoor air is used to monitor the temperatures of both air and compost during the outline of harvest time. The carbon dioxide given off by the rising mycelium is also replaced by outdoor air. The more mycelial growth, the more carbon dioxide produced, and since more growth occurs early in the yield, the more fresh air is required during the two breaks that underlie it. Likewise, the amount of fresh air depends on the growing mushrooms, the area of the distribution floor, the amount of compost provided in the growing room and the state or piece of fresh air. Experience is apparently the best guide on the volume of air required, but there is a general guideline: 0.3ft / hour when the compost is 8 inches deep, and 50 to 100 percent of this volume must be outside air.

A question often arises about the need for enlightenment while the mushrooms grow. Mushrooms do not need light to grow, photosynthesis requires light only from green plants. Growing rooms can be illuminated to promote harvesting or cropping activities, but it is more popular for staff or mushroom farmers to be furnished with miner's lamps instead of lighting a whole house.

Ventilation is important for growing mushrooms, and humidity and temperature controls are also required. A cold mist or live steam may add humidity to the air, or simply by wetting the walls and floors. Moisture can be removed from the growing room by: 1) allowing for a larger volume of outdoor air; 2) introducing drier air; 3) moving the same amount of outdoor air and heating it up to a higher temperature, as warmer air holds more moisture and thus lowers relative humidity. Control of temperature in a mushroom growing room is no different from control of temperature in your home. Heat can come from hot water that circulates through pipes that are mounted on walls. In recent mushroom farms, hot, forced air can be blown through a ventilation duct, which is rather common. There are a few mushroom farms in limestone caves where, depending on the time of year, the rock serves as both a heating and cooling surface. Caves of any kind are not necessarily suitable for growing mushrooms, and abandoned coal mines have too many intrinsic problems for a mushroom farm to be considered viable sites. Only calcareous caves require extensive reconstruction and enhancement before they are suitable for growing mushrooms, and only the growth occurs in the cave where composting takes place at a wharf above ground.

Mushrooms are harvested in a 7-to 10-day cycle, but this may be longer or shorter depending on the temperature, moisture, cultivar and the stage when they are picked. Once picking mature mushrooms a mushroom growth inhibitor is eliminated and the next flush progresses towards maturity. Mushrooms are usually picked at a time when the veil isn't stretched too far. Consumers in North America want mushrooms closed, tight, while flat mushrooms are wanted open in England and Australia. A mushroom's maturity is assessed by how far the veil is stretched, and not by how big the mushroom is. Consequently, mature mushrooms are both large and small, although both farmers and consumers prefer mushrooms of medium to large size.

Methods of picking and packaging also differ between farms. Freshly harvested mushrooms must be kept at 35° to 45° F for refrigeration. It is vital that mushrooms "breathe" after harvest to extend the shelf-life of the mushrooms, so storage in a non-waxed paper bag is preferred to a plastic bag.

The growing room should be closed off after the last flush of mushrooms has been collected, and the room should be pasteurized with steam. This final pasteurization is designed to destroy any pests that may be present in the growing room in the crop or woodwork, thereby minimizing the likelihood of infesting the next crop.

Conclusion

It takes about 15 weeks to complete a complete production cycle, from the beginning of composting to the final steaming off after harvesting has finished. A mushroom grower should expect from 0 to 4 lbs. in any position for this job. The national average for 1980 was 3.12 lbs. per square foot; Every Foot Square. Final yield depends on how well a grower has controlled the temperature, humidity, pests, etc. All things considered, the most significant factors for good production appear to be experience plus an intuitive feel for the commercial mushroom's biological rhythms. After the fundamentals of mushroom growth are known, the production system used to grow a crop can be selected.

www.ingramcontent.com/pod-product-compliance
Lightning Source LLC
Chambersburg PA
CBHW052345220526
45465CB00003BA/966